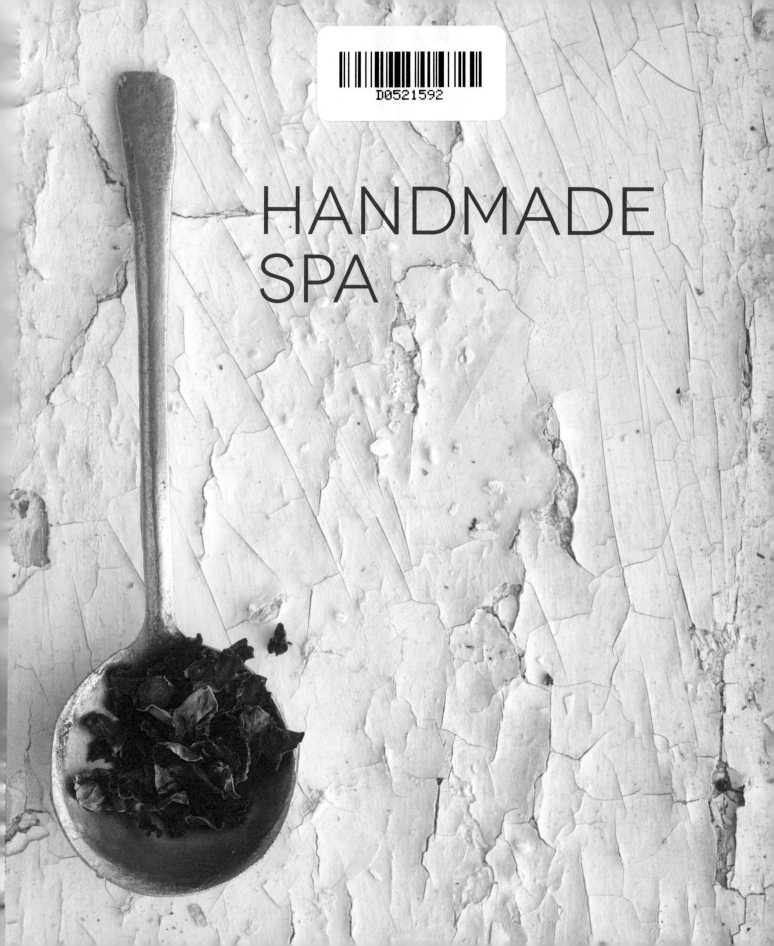

HANDMADE SPA

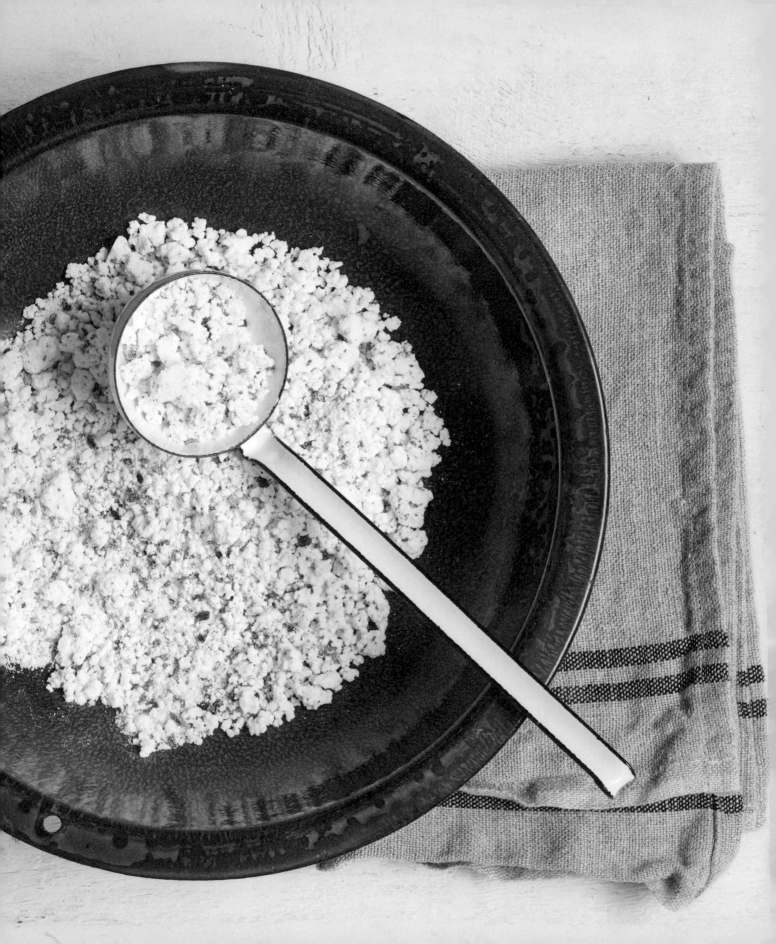

HANDMADE
SPA NATURAL TREATMENTS TO REVIVE AND RESTORE

JULIETTE GOGGIN
AND ABI RIGHTON

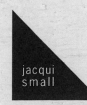

jacqui
small

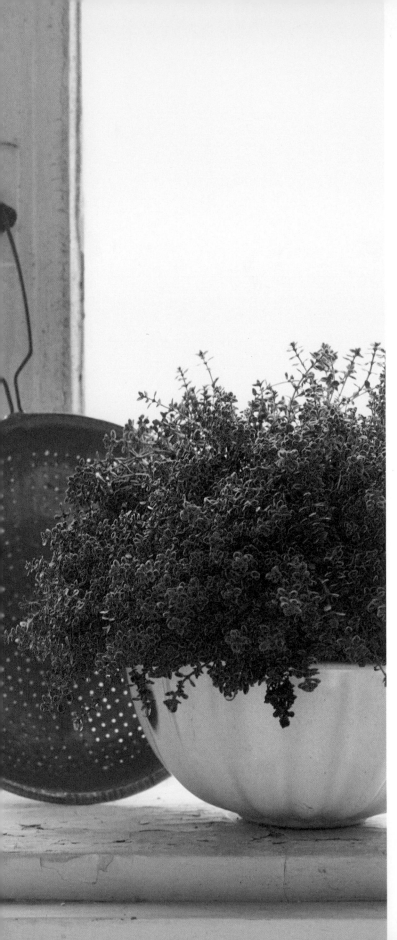

Design, layout and photography copyright ©
2018 Quarto Publishing Group plc
Text copyright © Juliette Goggin and Abi Righton

First published in 2018 by Jacqui Small
an imprint of The Quarto Group
The Old Brewery, 6 Blundell Street
London N7 9BH, United Kingdom
T (0)20 7700 6700 F (0)20 7700 8066
www.QuartoKnows.com

Publisher: Jacqui Small
Senior Commissioning Editor: Eszter Karpati
Managing Editor: Emma Heyworth-Dunn
Design and Art Direction: Rachel Cross
Editor: Rachel Malig
Photographer: Amanda Heywood
Stylist: Caroline Davis
Production: Maeve Healy

ISBN: 978 1 91112 719 2

A catalogue record for this book
is available from the British Library.

2020 2019 2018
10 9 8 7 6 5 4 3 2 1

Printed in China

Please note that the cosmetic industry is highly regulated and commercial
products undergo extensive trials and testing to ensure their long shelf-life and
safety. It is therefore important to understand that the recipes described in this
book are intended for the home crafter and not for selling on to the public.

Quarto is the authority on a wide range of topics.
Quarto educates, entertains and enriches the lives of
our readers – enthusiasts and lovers of hands-on living.

www.QuartoKnows.com

CONTENTS

Introduction

There's nothing better than the feeling of calm, relaxation and rejuvenation brought on by a luxurious, therapeutic spa session. From a simple pedicure, facial or massage at a high-street salon, to a state-of-the-art treatment featuring the latest therapies at a five-star spa hotel – all use a wide variety of products, ingredients and applications, and are designed to promote a feeling of health and well-being.

THE HISTORY OF THE SPA

Spa therapies are not a new trend and, like the use of essential oils and fragrance, can be traced back centuries.

The Ancient Greeks were one of the first documented, around 500BC, as using water from natural springs for therapeutic purposes, a practice embellished by the Romans with the creation of their incredibly ornate thermal baths at the sites of mineral and thermal springs. These were valued so highly that they were eventually built across the Roman Empire. As a result, thermal baths came to feature in the cultures of many countries around the world, and as the bathhouses developed, so too did the rituals surrounding them, to include massage and treatments based around steam and heat. These treatments were also enhanced by the use of essential oils and herbal teas.

In the Ottoman Empire, the hammam, or Turkish bath, took their inspiration from Ancient Rome. These bathhouses were open to everyone and served as a communal meeting place. A vigorous exfoliating scrub combined with steam was followed with a body wash and massage.

Some of these spas still exist today. In Istanbul and Marrakesh, stunning, ornate buildings have survived, and provide the authentic Turkish bath experience for both locals and tourists alike.

In Nordic countries, the spa tradition was based on extremes of hot and cold to boost the circulation. A sauna, featuring intense heat and steam, relaxed the body. Then a scrub with honey and sea salt was followed by lightly beating the skin with birch and eucalyptus twigs, and finally a dip in a plunge pool of cold water really kick-started the circulation, resulting in a sensation of exhilaration and well-being.

The spas of today are luxurious and bespoke, as increasingly people seek out experiences to help them relax, restore and rebalance the mind and body. Yet many of the old traditions continue, with the use of exfoliating, steam and massage treatments found in even the most ultra-modern, luxury spas, indicating that the ideas and influences of the past are still going strong.

THE HOME SPA

In *Handmade Spa* we want to encourage you to recreate the spa experience at home, using recipes you have made yourself and tailored to your own particular needs, so you can enjoy that feeling of well-being, relaxation and luxury as often and as easily as you wish.

Our passion is to create natural recipes and therapies using simple, easy-to-obtain ingredients, which can be

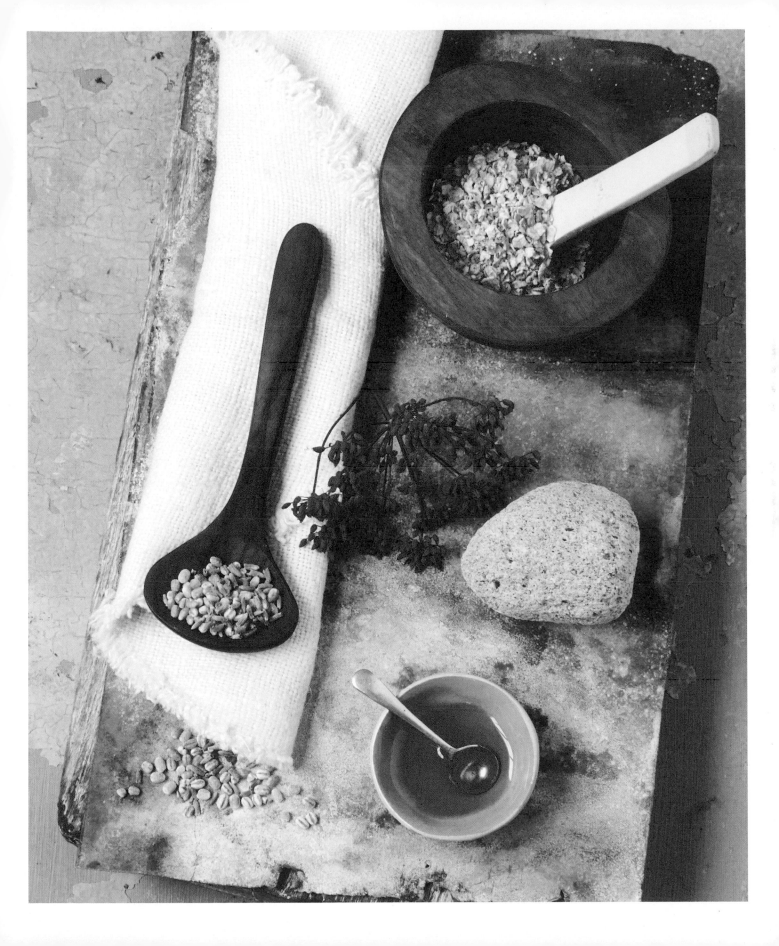

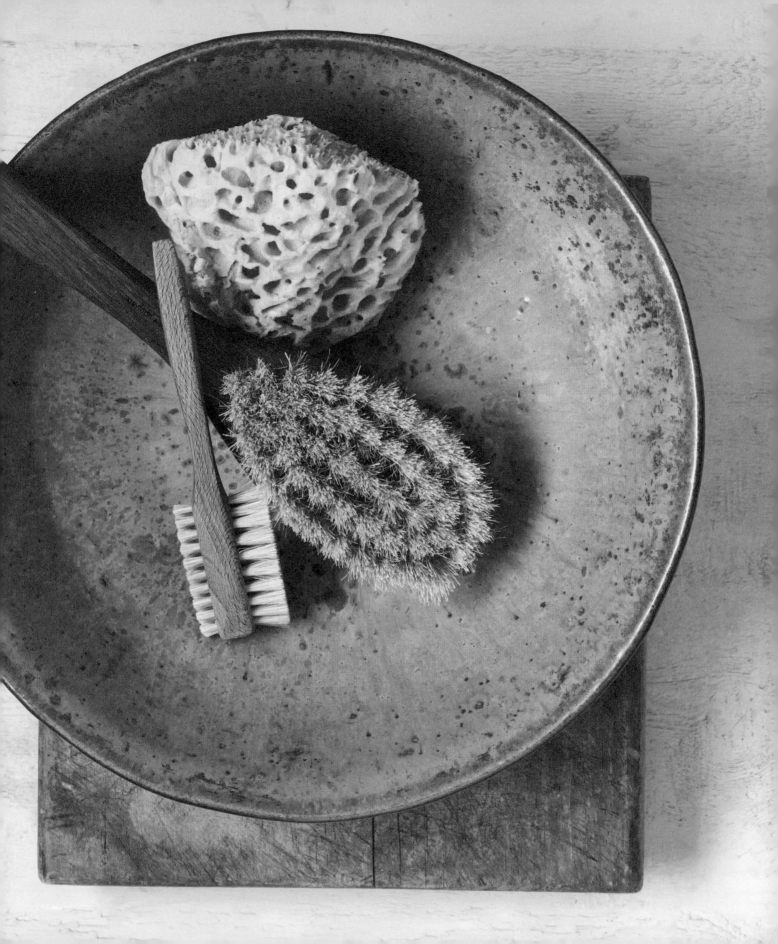

replicated at home. In this book we focus on treatments and associated recipes that reflect this ethos, harnessing the benefits of plants from the garden and herbs from the kitchen, combined with simple techniques to enable you to create your own products – both fresh ones to try straight away, and those you can store for future use to prolong that spa experience and enjoy additional benefits.

We have arranged the recipes in the book into chapters based on the differing properties of the scents and oils used: whether you want to be energized, comforted and warmed, regenerated and balanced, relaxed or detoxed, there is a recipe for you. You will find products for use on the body, face and hair, including cleansers, masks, scrubs, soaps, bath tablets, face and body creams, and a refreshing eau de toilette, as well as more therapeutic products, such as candles, herbal teas, reed diffusers and pillow mists, to create a truly holistic experience.

We also focus on key techniques, giving you the inside knowledge on how to create a salon-style hot cloth cleanser, and detailed instructions on how to make a variety of eye-catching candles and mood-enhancing incense products. A section on massage tips will also help you to work on soothing some of those aching muscles.

And we haven't forgotten the importance of preparing your surroundings so that your spa experience is maximized. We have provided numerous tips on how to set the desired atmosphere, discussing the importance of soft lighting, the right fluffy towels and the benefits of many other helpful accessories. Whether you want to be revived and energized or sent off to a blissful sleep, you can create the environment, recipes and associated scents to do so.

FRAGRANCE FAMILIES

Fragrance is a bit of a mysterious world – difficult to explore, to discover, and to find your own style. A basic understanding of the way in which fragrances are grouped into families will help you navigate your way around this fascinating world and hopefully make choosing what you want, or what you need, just a little easier.

The idea of using fragrances and perfumery has been around for thousands of years, from the earliest examples of aromatic plants, woods and tree resins such as frankincense and myrrh being burned over fire to cleanse and scent the air, to the Ancient Egyptians' use of scented oils and balms for burial purposes. Over time, the use of oils, herbs and fragrant plants became more widespread for therapeutic purposes, and also in perfumes for the body and to scent the home, much as we do today through the use of candles and reed diffusers.

'Modern' perfumery began in Italy and France, where the warm climate suited the growing of scented, aromatic plants such as rose, violet, lavender and jasmine. The French town of Grasse became the home of high-quality natural aromatic ingredients and also developed many of the techniques that led to the creation of perfumery as we know it today, including the introduction of new, synthetic ingredients which vastly increased the perfumer's creative options. Most famous of all was the creation of the iconic Chanel No 5 in 1921, which used an accidental overdose of chemicals called aldehydes to give a revolutionary and exciting top note to floral fragrances.

As the fragrance business became established, it was decided to categorize perfumes into families, and broadly speaking this has continued, as it enables experts to describe, reference and organize fragrances. Of course, fine fragrance, as eau de toilettes and perfumes are generally known, involves the blending of natural essential oils as well as synthetic ingredients to enable the perfumer to create perfumes around complex fragrance notes that do not exist as natural ingredients. It also allows the creator to make much cheaper fragrances than if they used entirely natural ingredients.

There are two means of cataloguing fragrance: the genealogy chart or the fragrance wheel. The best known and probably the easiest to follow is the Haarmann and Reimer Genealogy Chart. No longer in print, it is possible to find this online, and it categorizes perfumes into three distinct groups.

ESSENTIAL OILS

We use entirely natural essential oils to create the scents in our spa treatments. This type of blending of essential oils owes more to the field of aromatherapy, where the natural essential oils are used for their therapeutic qualities as much as their scent. Such products are simpler than fine fragrances, but can be similarly categorized in terms of scent, and the associated therapeutic and health benefits.

Refreshing, Revitalizing, Uplifting

Citrus oils are known for their refreshing, cleansing and revitalizing qualities. These are great to use in products to wake you up and refresh you when you're hot and tired. Examples include sweet orange, grapefruit, lime, lemon, bergamot and mandarin, which relate to some of the fragrances found in the Green, Fresh and Fruity family. We have also added herbal oils such as mint, marjoram and basil, as well as fresh floral notes from melissa and neroli.

Warming, Relaxing, Soothing

This section is all about comforting and soothing the body and mind, and we have used a combination of essential oils predominantly from the Woody and Floral families. The rich, spicy and woody essences of ginger, cedarwood, cinnamon, frankincense and sandalwood are warming to the skin, and have long-lasting qualities when used in home fragrance products such as candles. Other beneficial oils that could be used are from herbs such as lavender, thyme, clary sage and chamomile, together with floral oils such as ylang ylang, geranium and jasmine.

Regenerating, Balancing

This chapter is primarily based around flowers and uses their regenerating and balancing qualities to produce restorative treatments. They relate most directly to the Floral families, with some Fruity notes. As many floral essential oils are extremely rare and expensive, the selection is smaller than the other chapters, and key oils include rose, ylang, palmarosa, neroli, jasmine and geranium, as well as sweet orange and frankincense to give depth.

Calming, Restful, Sleep-Inducing

This section relates mostly to Floral and Woody families. We use herbs such as lavender, valerian and chamomile, which are well known for their relaxing and sleep-inducing qualities, as well as hops. Juniper, marjoram and clary sage are also represented, along with sandalwood and rose.

Detoxifying, Cleansing

The recipes here use fresh elements from citrus ingredients for their cleansing properties, as well as seaweed, roots and herbs known for their detoxifying properties. These are associated with the Green, Fresh and Fruity family, and key oils include lemongrass, lemon balm, peppermint, fennel, juniper, ginger and cedarwood.

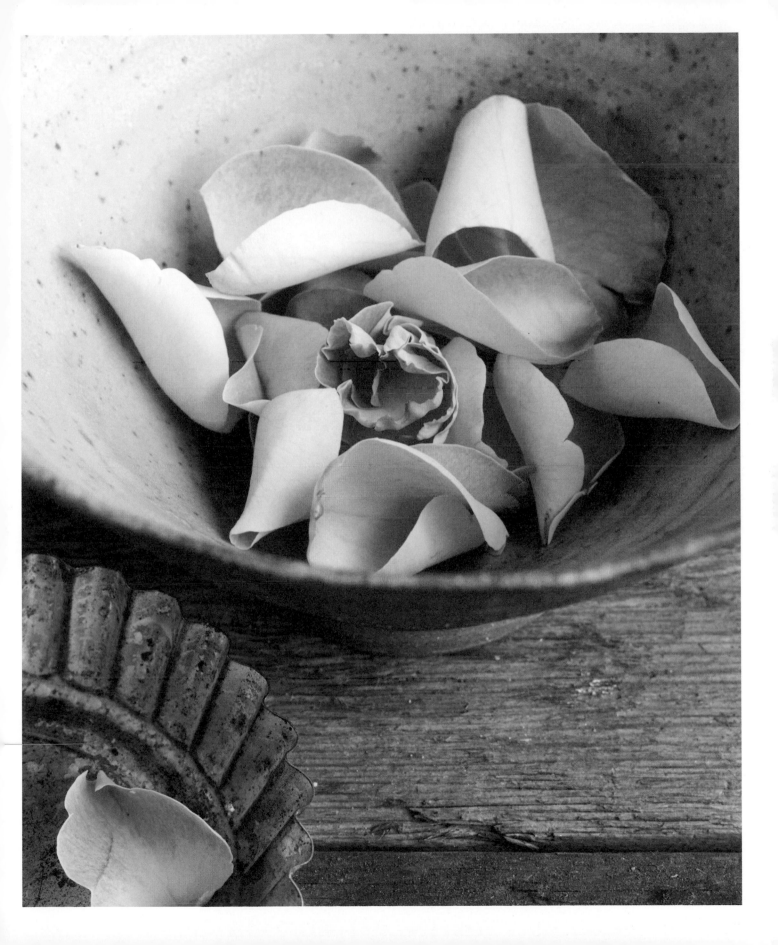

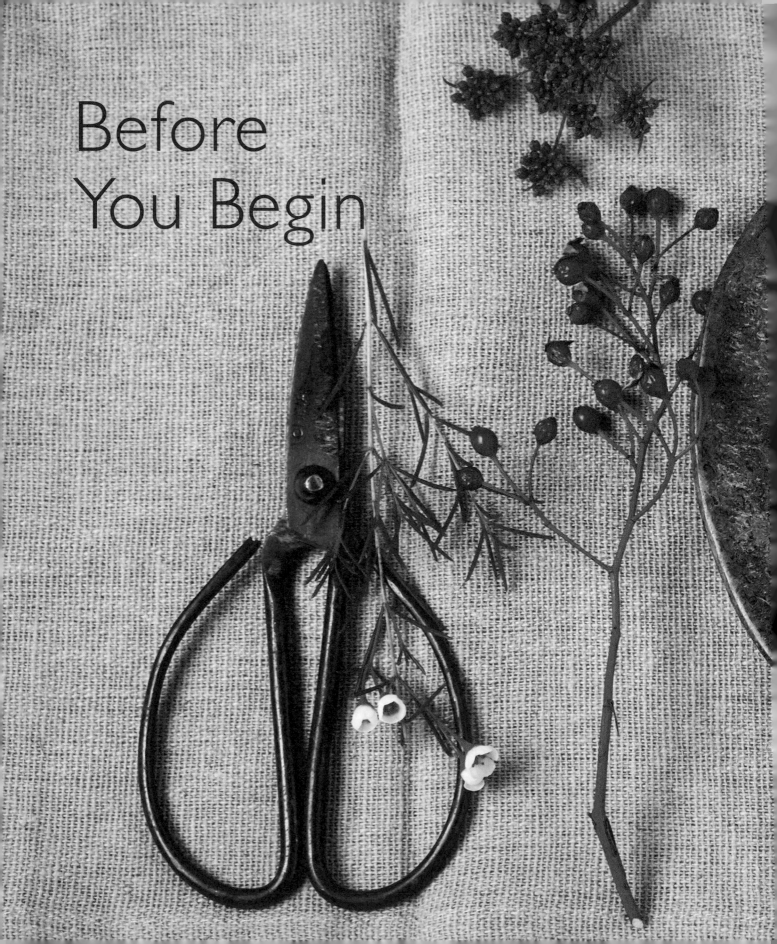

Before
You Begin

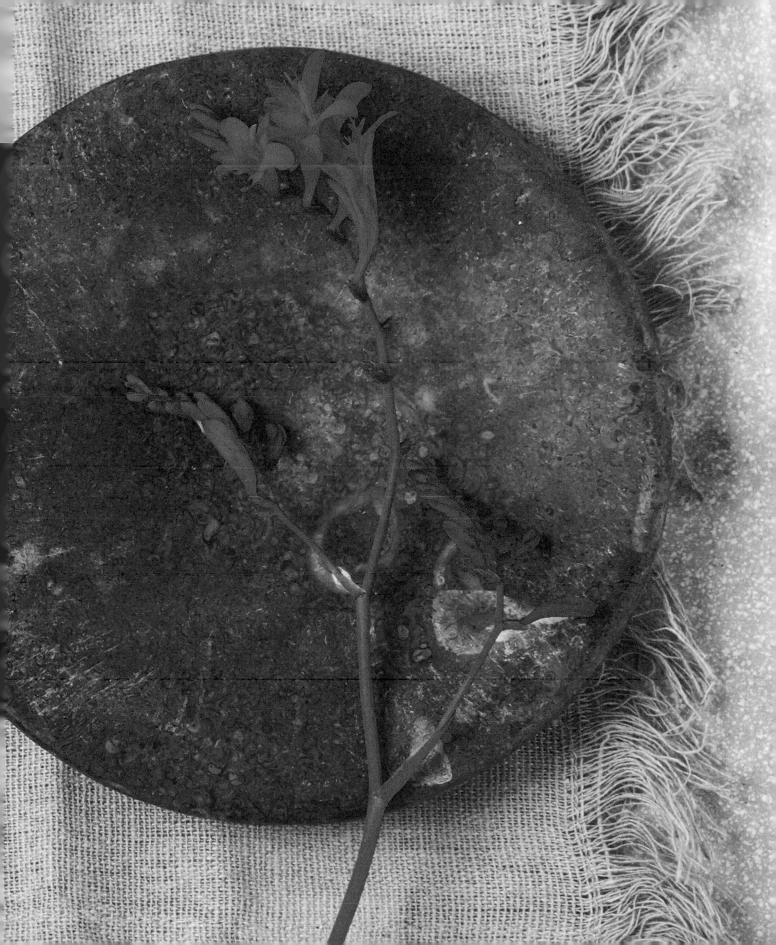

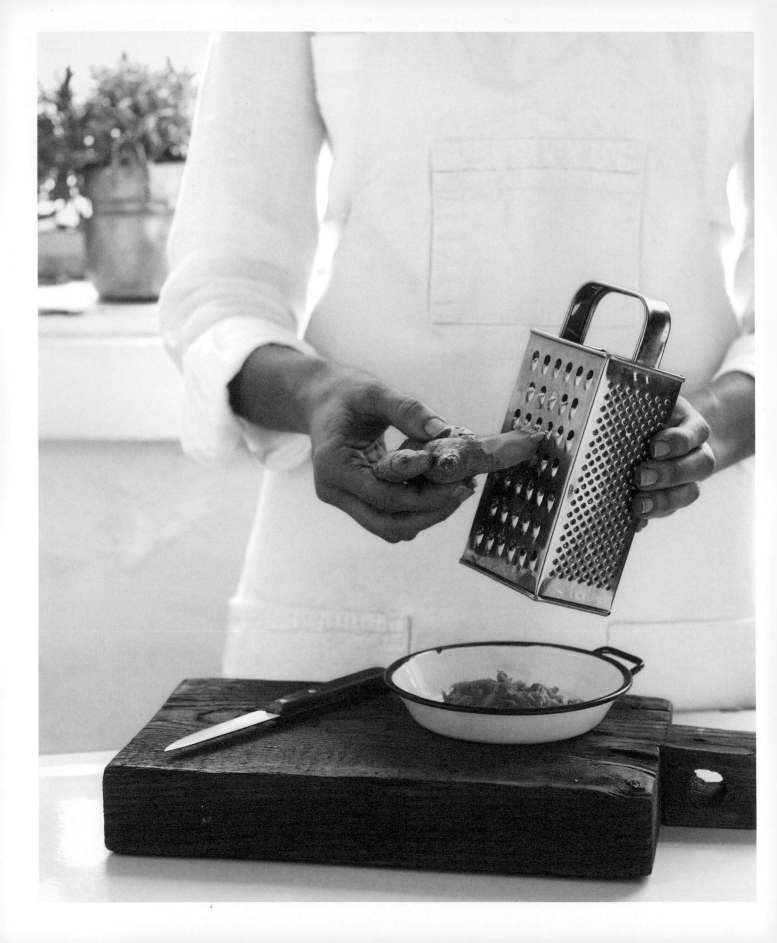

Preparing Your Ingredients

FINDING THE INGREDIENTS FOR YOUR SPA PRODUCTS IS EASIER THAN YOU MIGHT THINK. TAKE INSPIRATION FROM THE FLOWERS AND HERBS IN YOUR GARDEN, OR THE FRUIT AND VEGETABLES IN THE SUPERMARKET. PERHAPS YOU ALREADY USE ESSENTIAL OILS, OR SEE THEM IN YOUR LOCAL HEALTH-FOOD STORE. EVERYDAY THINGS WILL INSPIRE YOU TO GET CREATIVE, AND BEFORE YOU KNOW IT, YOU WILL BE READY TO TRY YOUR FIRST RECIPE.

In the Home

SEARCH YOUR CUPBOARDS

You will be surprised just how many of the items needed for the recipes in this book can already be found in your own home. A quick search through your kitchen and bathroom cupboards may reveal a few gems which can be put to an alternative use in your home spa.

- **Cellulose gum:** Commonly used for sugar work in cake decorating, this ingredient is excellent as a thickener in body washes and bath soaks. It also serves as a binder in our Incense Cones (see page 120).
- **Citric acid:** Used in jam-making as a preservative, citric acid also has cleaning properties so it is a useful kitchen cupboard item. Citric acid is a key ingredient in our Detoxifying Fizzing Seaweed Bath Tablets (see page 108), enabling the product to fizz when combined with sodium bicarbonate and water.
- **Fruits and vegetables:** Fruits and vegetables, such as cucumber and root ginger, are used in several of our recipes.

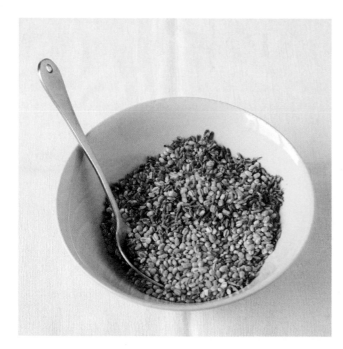

- **Gelatine:** We use a vegetarian and vegan gelatine in our recipes. If you also prefer to use non-animal products, be sure to check the manufacturer's ingredient list carefully. Gelatine is available as a clear sheet or as a powder version, which we use for our Cooling Cucumber, Matcha and Lime Face Mask (see page 42).
- **Glycerine:** This slightly syrupy liquid is frequently used as a cosmetic ingredient due to its ability to hold moisture to the skin. Beneficial herbs, roots, flowers and even seaweed can be steeped in a preserved glycerine and water mix to provide a range of naturally active ingredients for adding to creams and lotions.
- **Grains:** Rice and pearl barley are relatively inexpensive kitchen cupboard staples, and both form the filler for our Hot or Cold Soothing Wheat Pack (see page 64).
- **Herbal teas:** Green tea, either in leaf teabag or powder form, can be used as the basis of a water phase in some of the recipes, such as the Hot Cloth Facial Cleansers (see page 54) and Green Tea Eye Pads (see page 116).
- **Oils:** Olive oil, sunflower oil and rice bran oil can be found in most kitchens, and are cheap and versatile ingredients which can be used as a base oil for massage, or as an emollient in creams and lotions.
- **Porridge oats:** This breakfast staple is also known for its skin-soothing properties, and we use it in our Shower Mud with Juniper, Cypress and Fennel (see page 110).
- **Sea salt:** Sea salt contains a high level of naturally occurring minerals and is both detoxifying and exfoliating to the skin; it can be added to baths or used in body and hand scrubs. In contrast, refined salt loses many of these trace elements in processing. Epsom salts differ from sea salt in that they are a pure compound of magnesium and sulphate, but they also have numerous health and skincare benefits, and we use them in our Sauna Face Mask with Frankincense and Cypress (see page 52).
- **Spices:** Some well-known spices such as cinnamon and star anise are useful for preparing herbal teas.
- **Stevia:** This natural sugar substitute is used as an exfoliant

in our Mint Lip Scrub (see page 44), and also for its sweet flavour.

- **Unrefined coconut oil:** This ingredient has become very popular and much more widely available since its inclusion in many contemporary food recipes, and the discovery of its reputed health benefits. We like to use it in lip and foot scrubs as well as balms.
- **Witch hazel:** Traditionally used for treating insect bites, stings and minor irritations, witch hazel is a staple of the bathroom cupboard. It has so many uses in cosmetics due to its astringent properties, hence its inclusion in facial toners and cooling foot sprays. It also helps our Detoxifying Fizzing Seaweed Bath Tablets (see page 108) to stick together.
- **Xanthan gum:** A natural food thickening additive derived from corn sugar, which is often used in gluten-free recipes. We use xanthan gum to thicken and stabilize cosmetic creams and lotions. Premixing it with glycerine makes it easier to disperse in water.

USE THE INTERNET

It is almost impossible to imagine writing a specialist book such as *Handmade Spa* without the use of the internet. The ability to order products at the click of a mouse from the comfort of your home enables you to get started quickly, and to source some of the more specialist ingredients you may not already own.

For those slightly trickier ingredients you can't find in your home cupboards, you might be lucky enough to have a local ethnic grocer or health-food shop where you can source some of the floral waters and essential oils that we recommend, but you will also require some materials that are only available via online suppliers. Primarily, the internet will provide the more specialized items on your shopping list: preservatives, emulsifiers, oils and butters. They will also have a wider selection of essential oils than the health-food stores, but always check the pricing as regular deals on the high street can mean that they are cheaper on the more common items. Online sites are also the best place to search for containers for all the products you might wish to make, from jars for creams and scrubs, to bottles for lotions, shampoos and washes, as well as very small bottles, jars and pots for facial cleansers, serums and eye creams.

In recent years the rise in small-scale cosmetic and skincare companies has encouraged the growth of online suppliers of the very ingredients and equipment that those start-up companies require. This has also been a great help for the amateur maker. Eager to satisfy both markets, these companies provide a wide array of materials and equipment, as well as packaging. Some also offer tuition in the form of courses and classes and provide a few basic recipes for the beginner.

Like all things online, it is easy to get carried away, so do ensure that you check exactly what you need before ordering. The range is vast and it is easy to be tempted by a lovely sounding name without having a clear idea of what you might do with it. The likelihood is that after a few months it will still be waiting for that special project. You will also find that raw material ingredients are cheaper in bulk amounts, but be aware that they do have a shelf life, and most internet companies have an additional charge for postage which is generally based on weight, so it is sensible to buy only what you think you need for the recipes you are planning now.

The internet is also a way of finding other like-minded people with whom you can exchange ideas. Some of the social media sites such as Facebook and Instagram have groups you can join, giving the opportunity to swap ideas, air experiences and problems with both amateurs and professionals, and maybe find some new friends at the same time.

See the Directory of Suppliers on page 142 for a detailed list of online suppliers of a wide range of products used throughout the book. Details are given for a number of suppliers worldwide, and many offer both local and international shipping options. Hopefully you will find what you are looking for!

In the Garden

Many of us have discovered the joy of growing our own plants and flowers in gardens, courtyards, patios or window boxes. It is surprising what can be achieved with a bit of planning in even the smallest of spaces.

You may have thought about growing vegetables or some herbs for cooking, but we would love to encourage you to think about adding a few more plants for use in cosmetic recipes to enhance your home spa experience. The opportunity to pick your own herbs and flowers will inspire and enrich your recipes with the freshest and most potent of ingredients, grown in your own back garden and at your fingertips whenever you need them.

BENEFICIAL HERBS

A selection of herbs such as lemon balm, sage, mint, marjoram, camomile, lavender, fennel, pelargonium (also known as rose geranium) and thyme are used in many of the recipes. Fresh herbs can be used in herbal teas and facial steams, but for wheat packs, incense, bath oils, powders and herb pillows, dried herbs are required. Simply place your fresh herbs in an airing cupboard on a paper-lined tray and they will dry within a few days. Keep them in airtight containers in a cool, dry place until required.

BENEFICIAL FLOWERS

As well as herbs, try growing flowers such as healing calendula, St John's wort and achillea, immune-boosting echinacea, fragrant roses (flowers and rose hips) for cosmetics and teas, elderflowers for creams and lotions, hops to aid sleep, and violas and daisies for soothing balms.

Even unpopular weeds such as nettles can be useful for hair products. Or if you only have a windowsill, why not cultivate an aloe plant which will give you an instant cooling gel for treating sunburn and an all-purpose soothing skincare ingredient.

Only use flowers in perfect condition and fully open; avoid damaged petals or any that are imperfect in colour or shape. Also avoid any flowers or plants that are potential irritants or poisonous.

USING FLOWERS AND HERBS IN THE RECIPES

FOR THE DISPERSING BATH OIL *(page 74)*
Lavender, oregano, marjoram, rosemary, roses, calendula or late-flowering daisy-headed flowers such as echinacea and achillea are ideal for use in this oil.

FOR THE FACIAL STEAM WITH FLOWERS
(page 72) A facial steam is a great way to benefit from the power of soothing and healing plants. Try lavender, camomile, rose and calendula for their soothing and calming properties, or fennel, juniper, sage and thyme for problem skin.

FOR THE PURIFYING INCENSE POWDER
(page 118) For powder incense recipes you can add botanical ingredients to the mix of wood powders and resins which form the base. Try dried pelargonium leaves, sage, thyme or rosemary, dried pine needles, cistus and marjoram as well as lavender flowers.

FOR THE SLEEPY HERBAL AND DETOX TEAS
(pages 99 and 115) Rose petals, peppermint and spearmint leaves can be used fresh or dried in teas and infusions. Lime flowers from the linden tree can also be added if you are fortunate enough to have this majestic tree in your garden.

FOR THE CAMOMILE EYE PADS *(page 116)*
As well as using dried camomile tea, you could use fresh camomile flowers which have a stronger and much fresher aroma than dried flowers.

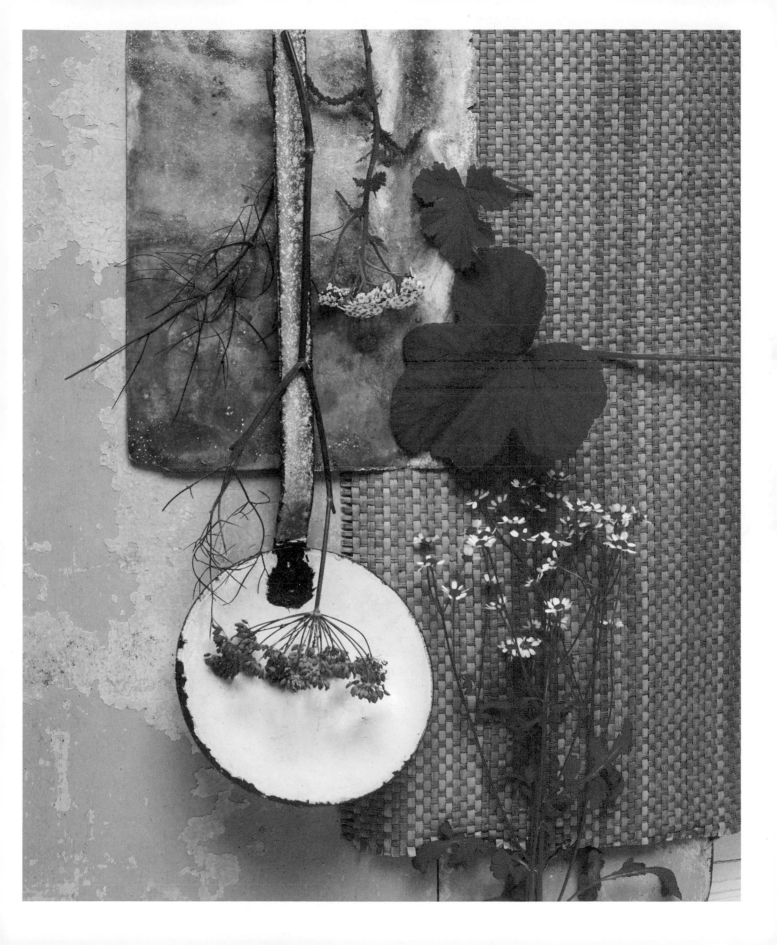

Essential Oils

Essential oils are volatile aromatic compounds extracted from fruits, flowers, leaves, woods and roots. They have a long history of use in aromatherapy, traditional medicines and cosmetic products, and have extraordinary powers which can be harnessed to give both a delightful and evocative scent as well as specific beneficial properties.

They are not to be confused with the natural vegetal oils, such as sweet almond or sunflower oil, which are usually cold-pressed from the kernel/nut or seed of the plant. Vegetal oils are not aromatic and only have a bland, mildly fatty scent, but their varying fatty acid profiles offer different therapeutic skincare benefits, including emollient and moisturizing properties.

Essential oils are obtained by one of three methods:

Steam Distillation

The most common method is steam distillation, in which the essential oil is obtained by infusing the plant material with steam. The high temperature releases the oils from the plant material, which are carried through with the steam to a condenser where the essential oil separates on to the surface of the water. Useful bi-products of this method are the flower water condensates such as rose, lavender and orangeflower, which we use extensively in our recipes. They contain the water-soluble aromatic fractions of the plant material and, although very much weaker than the corresponding essential oil, they still impart a delightful and characteristic scent when used to replace plain water in recipes. They are also excellent toners in their own right.

Solvent Extraction

The most expensive flower oils, such as rose and jasmine absolute, are obtained via solvent extraction, where the cut flowers are mixed with a solvent to 'dissolve' the essential oil from the plant, as well as the waxes present. This will firstly provide a 'concrete' or solid from which the absolute oil is obtained. The resulting oil, or absolute yield, is very low for these precious oils, for example 100kg (220lb) of rose petals can produce as little as 500ml (17fl oz) of essential oil. It's no surprise, therefore, that some oils can cost thousands of pounds per litre. Hence you will often find oils such as rose, jasmine and even chamomile sold as dilutions in very small bottles, typically 5–10 per cent in a carrier oil. It is important to check what dosage of oil you are buying, although the price will be a good indication.

Expression

Citrus oils are usually extracted via expression, which involves crushing the fruit to obtain the oil from the outer rind. The whole fruit can be used and the oil separated, or the peel can be used on its own. Oils produced via expression include sweet orange, grapefruit and lemon.

USING ESSENTIAL OILS

In *Handmade Spa* we have used essential oils both for their scent and their therapeutic qualities, and each chapter is based on a theme which relates very closely to the properties of the essential oils used. There are revitalizing citrus and herbal oils to refresh and uplift; warming and relaxing woody and spicy oils to comfort and soothe; balancing and regenerating floral oils such as ylang ylang, neroli and geranium; relaxing, sleep-promoting traditional herbal oils from lavender and hops; and detoxifying fennel and ginger and fresh, cleansing citrus and mint oils.

Essential oils are expensive, but are used in small quantities so a little goes a long way. Some general rules on dosage are that facial skincare products should contain no more than 0.5 per cent of essential oils. In leave-on body products, such as body lotions and creams, 1 per cent is generally sufficient, and in wash-off products such as body washes, bath essences and soaks, between 1 and 3 per cent is normal, depending on the strength of the individual oils.

The oils can last for a few years if they are well looked after. Do remember that these oils are delicate and can be adversely affected by external conditions, therefore they should be stored in amber glass bottles with a minimal 'head space' (air above the oil) and with tightly fitting lids to protect from light and oxidation. Store in cool temperatures – 8–20°C (46–68°F) is fine – to maximize shelf life.

ESSENTIAL OIL SAFETY

Essential oils are powerful ingredients and should be used with care. They should never be used directly on the skin as they can cause an allergic reaction in some people. They should also never be used in products for the eyes. Certain essential oils are contra-indicated for use in pregnancy, or for those with certain medical conditions, so they should be avoided in these cases.

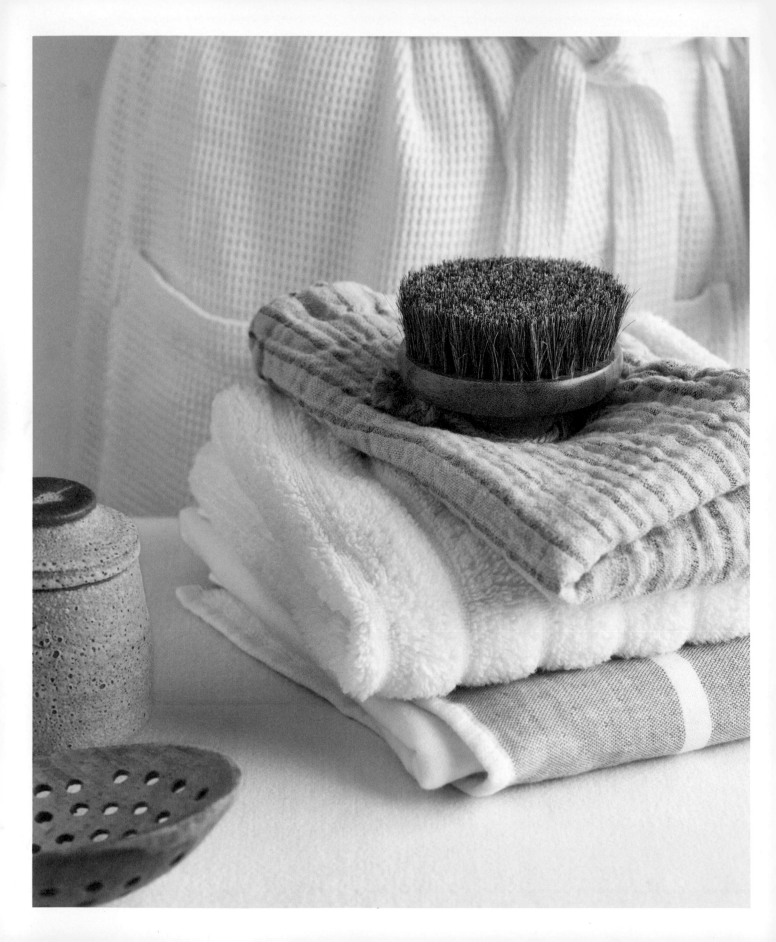

Preparing Your Spa

CREATING THE RECIPES IN THE BOOK REQUIRES VERY LITTLE IN THE WAY OF SPECIALIST ITEMS, AND MOST KITCHENS WILL HAVE ENOUGH OF THE BASICS TO GET YOU STARTED. YOU MAY NEED TO STOCK UP ON A FEW SPA TOOLS TO ALLOW YOU TO FULLY ENJOY THE TREATMENTS YOU MAKE. NATURAL INGREDIENTS REQUIRE CAREFUL PREPARATION AND STORAGE, SO DO FOLLOW OUR GUIDELINES CAREFULLY WHEN WORKING WITH THEM.

Equipment

Many of the cosmetic preparations in *Handmade Spa* resemble cookery recipes, so you will not be surprised to discover that most kitchens contain the tools required to make them. We have divided the equipment list into Basic and Specialist sections, so you can try out a few of the easier recipes without having to buy any extra equipment.

It is good practice to have all of your equipment to hand before you begin. It is helpful to have a few metal teaspoons available when stirring and spooning ingredients, as you will be surprised how many you use. It can also be useful to have more than one heatproof jug to hand for the recipes that require adding multiple ingredients at different stages, or a selection of small glass bowls and jugs for measuring the ingredients in advance. Accurate measuring is essential, and this requires a set of digital scales; however, as most domestic kitchen scales do not measure less than 1 or 2 grams, very small measuring spoons are also advisable.

Recipes that require heating will need a gas or electric hob (stove). Some materials need to be 'cooked' prior to use, and so an oven and a baking tray (cookie sheet) are required. Timing is important, so a kitchen timer or stopwatch on a mobile (cell) phone will help.

For the less straightforward recipes some additional equipment is required, although many kitchens will also have most of these items already. A coffee grinder, Nutribullet or smoothie maker is useful for chopping fresh herbs and dried materials into the small-sized particles needed. A stick blender is also required for many of the creams, serums and lotions, as well as some of the scrubs. A pestle and mortar is useful for grinding tablets.

A very small 50ml (1½fl oz) measuring glass is helpful when mixing powders into liquids, such as xanthan gum and cellulose gum. The handle end of a metal teaspoon is the best way to mix very small quantities such as these. Plastic or metal funnels make dispensing liquids easier and are used with filter papers for filtering some liquids. And where stronger liquid ingredients such as essential oils do not have a dropper top, a plastic pipette can be used as a dispenser. This is also useful for working with Sucragel.

BASIC EQUIPMENT

Baking tray (cookie sheet) • Chopping board • Digital scales • Glass beakers • Glass bowls • Grater • Heatproof jugs • Jars with lids • Kitchen timer/stopwatch • Knives • Scissors • Sieve • Small measuring spoons • Stainless steel spoons: teaspoons, tablespoons, and a long-handled sundae spoon is very useful for stirring in large heatproof jugs • Stainless steel saucepans • Teapot and strainer

SPECIALIST EQUIPMENT

Bain marie *(ideally two, for heating ingredients and candle-making)* • Candle and soap moulds • Coffee grinder • Coffee filter paper • Glass/plastic bottles with a variety of caps: *screw cap, pump dispenser, spray cap* • Glass or plastic funnels • Glass rod (or flat-bladed knife) • Kitchen blender • Large jug • Large glass or ceramic bowl • Metal pourer for candle wax • Pestle and mortar • pH strips • Plastic box and lid for incense drying • Plastic pipette • Spatula • Stick blender • Thermometer • Tweezers • Vinyl gloves • 50ml (1½fl oz) measuring glass

A large glass or ceramic bowl can be helpful to use as a water bath to cool down liquids quickly prior to adding the final ingredients. The bowl should be half-filled with very cold or iced water to quickly reduce the temperature of the liquid in the heatproof jug or bowl placed inside it. A plastic washing-up bowl would also be suitable.

Candle-making also requires its own, more specialist equipment in the form of moulds for floating candles (scented candles can be made in drinking glasses or other similar vessels), a metal pourer for wax and a bain marie.

Finally, jars, bottles and other containers with correctly fitting lids are essential for storing finished recipes.

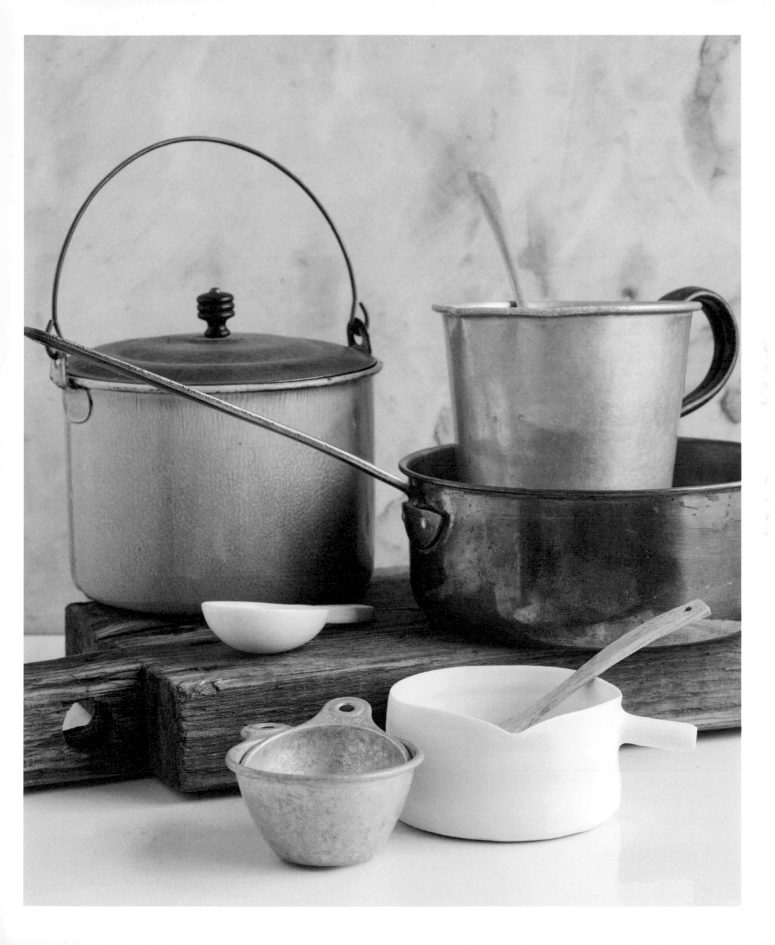

Spa Tools

A spa experience is something to treasure and remember; it's designed to linger in the memory and to entice you back when the pressures of everyday life seem just that bit too much.

SPA DESIGN

The design of the most prestigious spas is a highly specialized task, involving considerable experience and expense to create that very special ambience associated with a five-star day out. Recreating this in your own home requires a certain attention to detail, borrowing ideas from the experts to replicate the atmosphere of luxury, serenity and comfort.

Preparation and Planning

Spa treatments are associated with certain key tools, which might seem unimportant but which do make a difference: the most luxurious of deep-pile towels and soft, comforting waffle slippers really do enhance the treatments on offer and provide a sense of well-being that will seal the experience in your memory long after the day has passed. With some preparation and planning, you can ensure that your home spa is equipped with the correct tools and accessories to complement the wonderful natural recipes you have spent time creating.

SPA ACCESSORIES

In addition to the basic equipment needed for making the recipes themselves, you will need some or all of the following. You will almost certainly have many of them at home already, so it shouldn't be too tricky or expensive a task to collect them all together.

- **Wooden spatulas** for the application of muds and masks
- **Deep-pile towels** for body wraps and for the hair
- **Mitts** for body exfoliation or tanning application
- **Face cloths** for hot cloth facial cleansing and for removing face and body masks
- **Flat, round cellulose sponges** for removing face masks

- **Cotton wool pads** for cleansing
- **Pumice stones** for exfoliating
- **Bath lily** or natural sponges
- **Body brushes** to aid circulation and for anti-cellulite treatments
- **Loofah** for exfoliating
- **Orange sticks** and other manicure tools, such as nail brush, scissors, nail buffing tool, nail file
- **Massage roller** for body massage
- **Hairbands/hair clips** to be used for facials and face masks
- **Pillows** for supporting the body during massage and for general relaxation
- **Comfortable waffle slippers**
- **Blankets** for relaxation and for keeping the body warm and relaxed during treatments
- **Eye mask** for relaxation
- **Candles** or essential oil burners
- **Suitable music** can aid relaxation during treatments

It is a good idea to have a glass of water available after a treatment, as it will help to flush toxins from the body.

NATURAL SEA SPONGES

A natural sea sponge is a beautiful object with many unique properties, and ideal for your home spa. It can be used to gently exfoliate, to cleanse both body and face, to remove muds and masks, and even in massage techniques. Whether you're planning a revitalizing citrus shower scrub or a luxurious, relaxing soak in bath oil, make sure you have a natural sponge to hand for maximum skin-conditioning benefit. Natural sponges are easy to clean and, with care, will last much longer than synthetic, more abrasive sponges, making them a perfect, cost-effective spa accessory for the home.

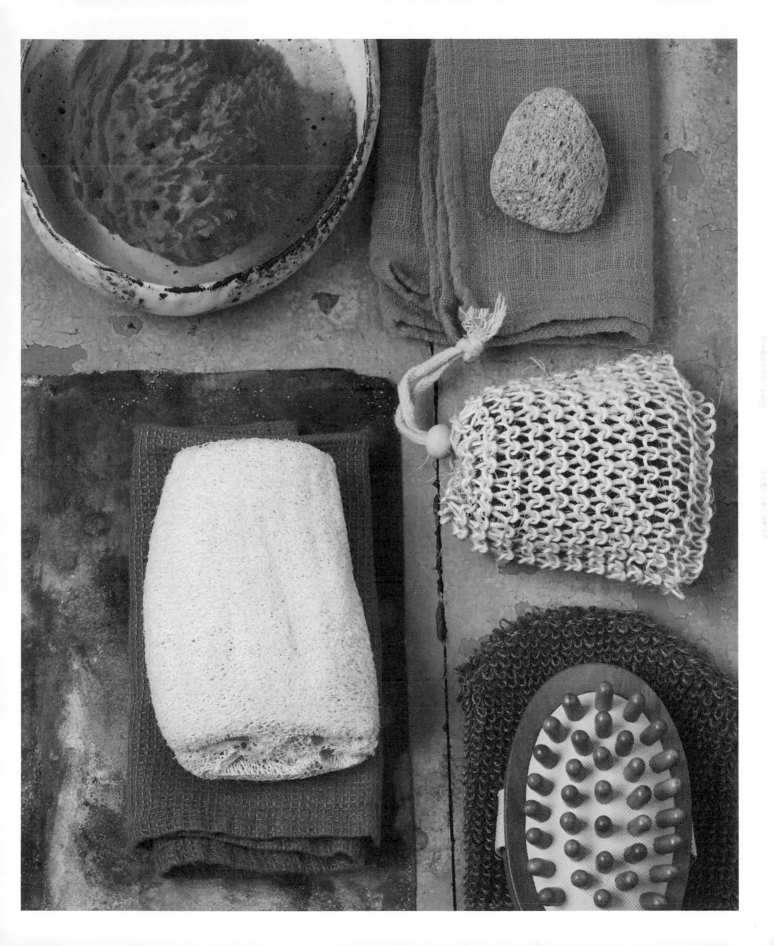

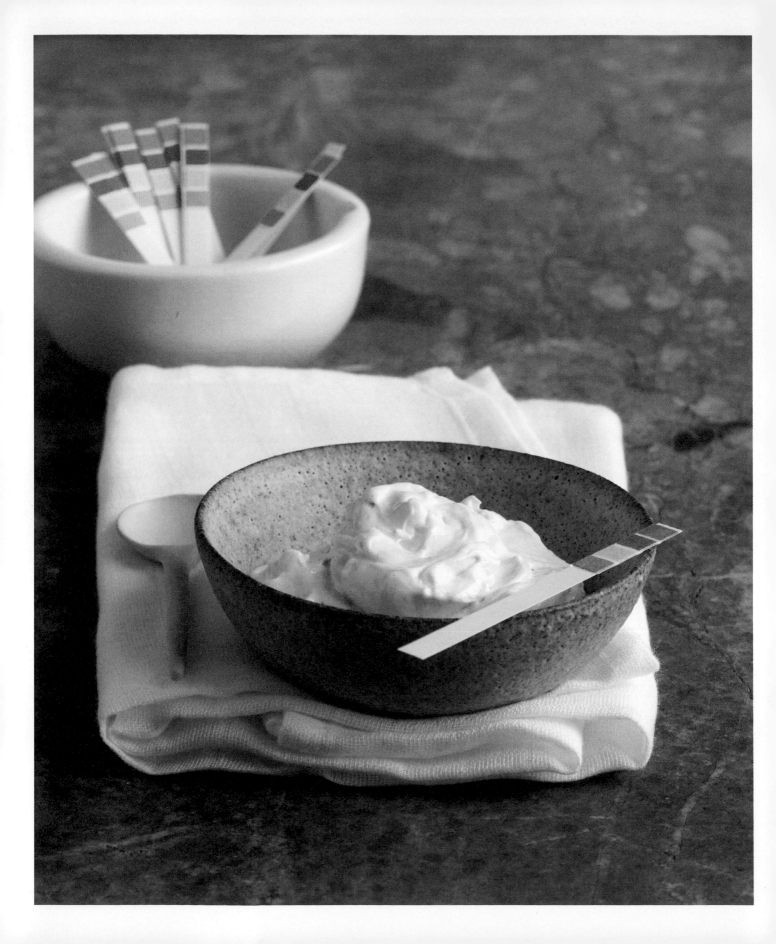

pH

Cosmetic products are designed to work in harmony with the natural balance of the skin, which helps to avoid undesirable skin irritations and allergic reactions. When preparing products for your home spa, it is important to create products which are gentle on the skin, and the pH is an indicator of this.

The pH of any substance is the measure of its acid or alkaline content and is ranked from 0 to 14, with pH 7, the natural acidity of water, being neutral. The further below 7 any value is, the more acidic it is, and the higher above 7 the more alkaline. The pH of healthy skin is 5.5, therefore most cosmetic products are formulated to be as close to this as possible, in order to feel comfortable and harmonious when in use.

Preservatives are effective only within specific pH bands, and it is therefore very important when using any preservative in a recipe to check its suitability and to use it within the band for which it is intended. This information should be provided with the product material when it is purchased, but if you are in any doubt at all, do double check with the supplier.

ALTERING THE PH OF A PRODUCT

The recipes in this book are designed to work within the required pH range that is suitable for the product and the preservative listed. However, should you need to reduce a pH, it can be done by the addition of a few drops of lactic, or citric acid solution. Add the solution gradually, stirring into the product to combine, and recheck the pH each time you do this. For wash products using Plantapon LGC, a natural foaming ingredient, and Lamesoft PO65, which is added for its moisturizing benefits, lowering the pH in this way to about 5.5 can help to increase the thickness and give a more professional edge to the products.

Any product that contains water requires a preservative if it is to be stored and not used immediately, so choosing the correct preservative is important. We indicate in each recipe if a preservative is required, so it is important to use one if we have listed it. The recipes in this book are chosen and tested to work with grapefruit seed extract, a natural preservative effective over a broad pH range, although it is most effective when used in a product with a pH of below 7.

MEASURING PH

There are several types of pH strip available online (see Directory of Suppliers, page 142). Having tried out a few different types we recommend the pH Indicator (0–14) Strips from Nova Health, or Universal pH Test Strips (0–14) from Simplex Health, both of which are easy to use and have clear instructions on the box.

Each strip is marked in sections with four coloured bands at one end. Each strip is identical and has the same coloured bands. The product box contains a picture of how the strips will appear once they have been used, and determining the final pH is a simple matter of matching the altered coloured strips with the coloured bands on the box and checking the pH number it corresponds to.

Using pH Strips

To test liquids or thin, pourable gels, dip a test strip into the liquid for around one second, then remove it from the product. Don't allow the strip to get too wet or the test squares may peel off. For creams or thicker lotions, press the strip down on to the surface of the product for 5 to 10 seconds, then carefully remove the strip from the surface to reveal the test squares.

Align the test strip with the coloured strips on the box and compare the two, checking the pH according to the new colours on the strip. The answer given will be within a small but allowable margin and is sufficient for home use. For total accuracy, a pH meter is the answer, but this is expensive and not generally required for personal use.

Storage and Safety

CARING FOR YOUR INGREDIENTS

- Buy ingredients from trusted sources. Store them in airtight containers in a cool, dry place away from sunlight, and mark with the date of purchase.
- Before using the ingredients, check that the appearance and odour is good. If the smell is 'off' or unpleasant, or if in doubt about the appearance, then discard.
- When handling and measuring out materials it is advisable to wear disposable gloves, especially when dispensing essential oils and surfactants. A face mask is advised if handling powders that are very dusty.
- Using deionized or demineralized water is preferable to using tap water in a recipe, as tap water contains traces of metal salts that may cause products to discolour. Always boil water before using to ensure sterility.
- When weighing materials, and mixing phases and batches, use only sterilized tools and vessels, and when transferring your product into containers, make sure the jars/bottles you are using are sterilized. Fill the containers to full capacity to avoid leaving too much 'head space' (air above the product) that will encourage oxidation.
- Natural ingredients can contain microbes that could be potentially harmful or spoil the finished product, so it's important that the ingredients used are properly prepared and treated to make them sufficiently sterile. Materials containing water such as flower waters and aqueous plant extracts are particularly vulnerable to microbes, but some materials which appear to be dry, such as flours or clays, can also contain sufficient moisture to harbour moulds. Carrier oils and essential oils do not contain water and are unlikely to carry microbes. The methods prescribed for the recipes in this book have been developed through trials and micro tests to give a sterile finished product. It is therefore very important that the methods are followed, especially where materials and phases require heating. Maintaining a minimum temperature of 70°C (158°F) for 30 minutes is the general rule to kill off most of the microbes, but for water-based products we have added a preservative to help keep contamination at bay and extend the product shelf-life. The ingredient that we have chosen to use to help preservation is grapefruit seed extract, which is readily available through internet cosmetic material suppliers. Waterless oil- and wax-based products such as massage oils and lip balms generally do not need preservatives to be added, but the addition of vitamin E can help against rancidity.
- Although many neat essential oils can be potentially irritating or sensitizing, if handled correctly the risks are much reduced. Dispense essential oils carefully, avoiding direct skin contact, and ensure that the area you are working in is ventilated. Take care not to get any around the eye. If this happens, rinse with plenty of cold water.

CARING FOR YOUR FINISHED PRODUCTS

- Store your products in a cool, dry place away from sunlight. Sunlight and heat are the worst for causing rancidity and degrading products. Mark the container with the date of preparation. Anhydrous, wax- or oil-based products can last for six months to a year, providing they are kept dry. Water-based products such as creams, lotions and toners should keep for three to six months, providing they are suitably preserved and the sterilizing and heating techniques are adhered to. Avoid dipping fingers into pots and leaving products exposed without lids, as microbes can be introduced.
- 'Fresh', unpreserved products should be kept in airtight containers in the fridge and used within two days.
- Always check your products before using them to make sure that the smell, colour and appearance is still good.
- Keep a log book containing details of each batch of product that you make, such as date of preparation and source of each ingredient. Note phase temperatures achieved and the length of time the temperature was maintained for. Note any variations that you may make from the book's recipes and methods. Check and record the pH of your water-based products using pH strips. If you notice differences in batches of the same product, the details in your log book may point to the reason.

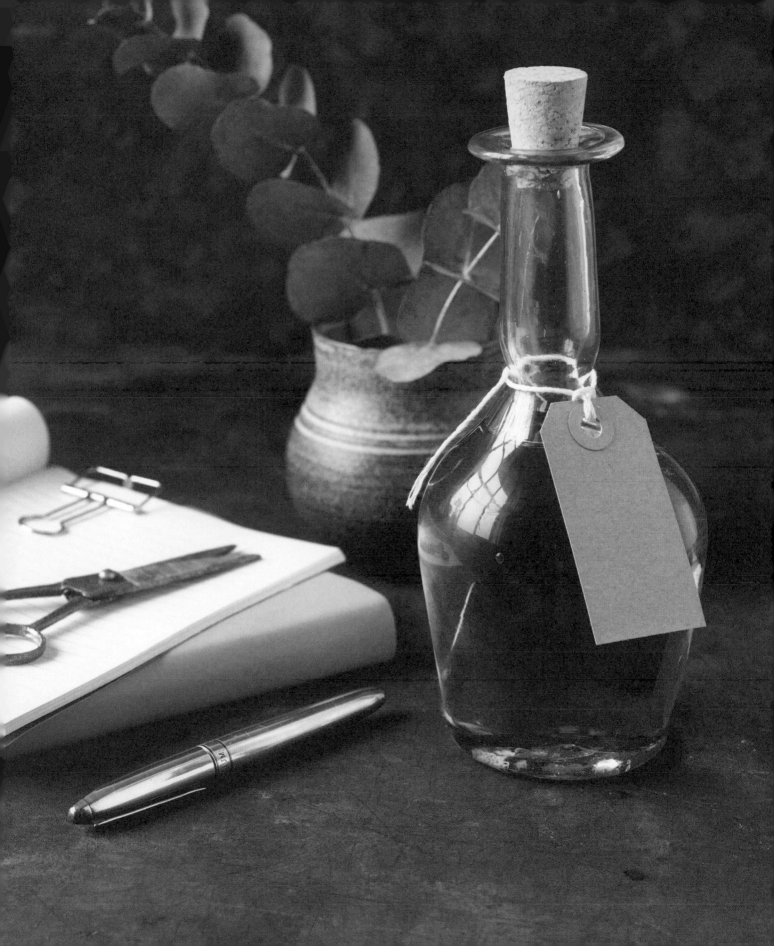

Product
Recipes

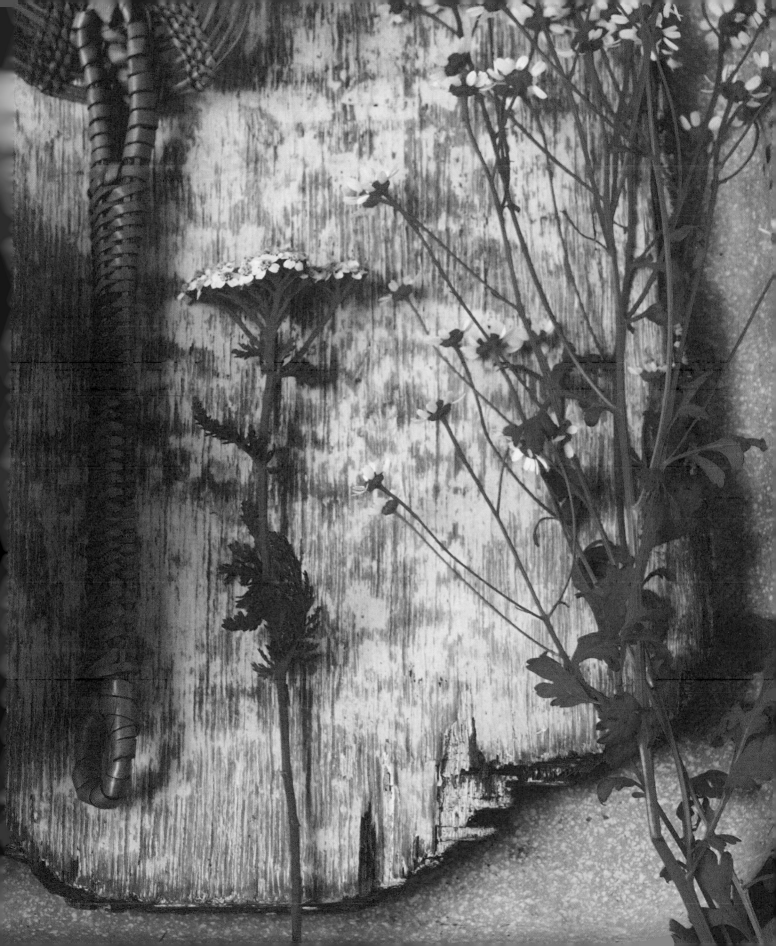

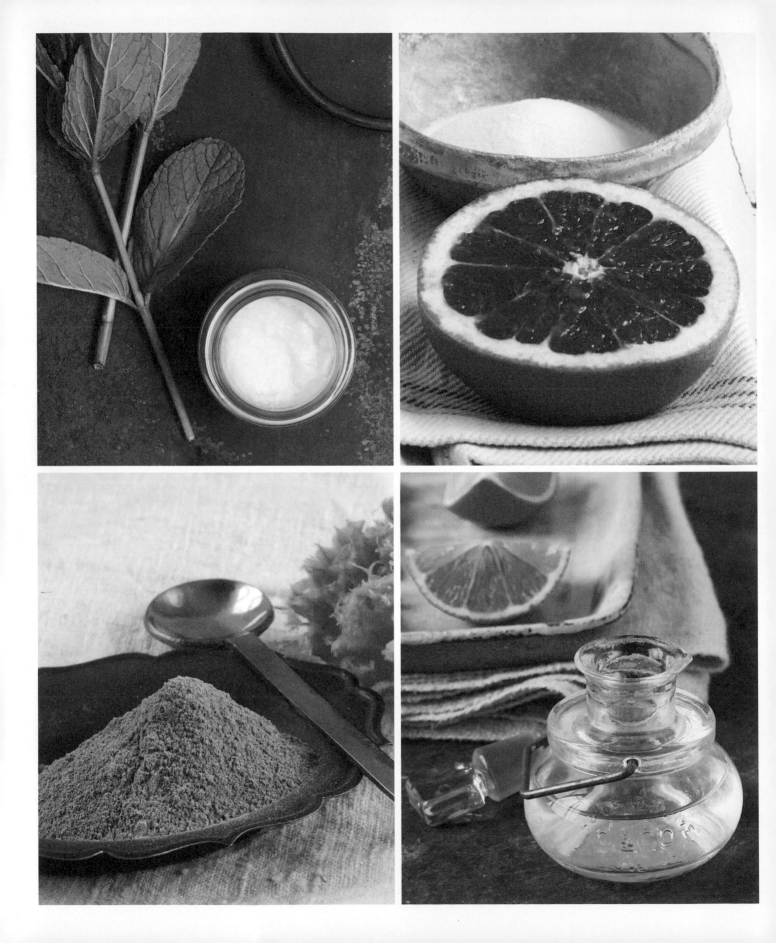

Refreshing, Revitalizing, Uplifting

REFRESHING AND REVITALIZING TREATMENTS ARE ASSOCIATED WITH CITRUS ESSENTIAL OILS, AND HERE YOU WILL FIND LEMON, SWEET ORANGE, GRAPEFRUIT, LIME, BERGAMOT AND MANDARIN, AS WELL AS HERBS SUCH AS MINT, ROSEMARY AND BASIL. UPLIFTING FLORAL ELEMENTS COME FROM NEROLI, AN ESSENTIAL OIL DERIVED FROM ORANGEFLOWER BLOSSOMS, AS WELL AS MELISSA, ALSO KNOWN AS LEMON BALM.

Revitalizing Facial Cleansing Grains

These cleansing grains contain antioxidant vitamin C and matcha green tea as well as dried lime powder to help brighten and polish the skin. The addition of Sucragel helps to disperse the grains while gently cleansing, leaving the skin feeling amazingly soft and smooth. Mixing the powder with a small amount of glycerine will add a moisturizing element to the cleansing treatment.

Makes approx. 100g (3½oz)

INGREDIENTS
40g (1½oz) green clay
39g (1½oz) porridge oats
3g (½ tsp) lime powder
  (dried Iranian limes)
5g (1 tsp) matcha green tea
  powder
1 x 4g vitamin C tablet (1000mg),
  or the equivalent in powder
8ml (1½ tsp) Sucragel CF
20 drops lemon essential oil

SPECIAL EQUIPMENT
baking tray (cookie sheet)
coffee grinder

SAFE STORAGE
Store in a cool, dry place, away from sunlight. Keeps for up to 3 months.

HOW TO APPLY
Place a small amount of the powder in the palm of one hand and add warm water to make a paste. Apply to the face and work into the skin with the fingertips. Wash off with plenty of warm water; a muslin cloth or small cellulose sponge is useful to help remove all traces of the cleansing grains. Alternatively, leave the cleanser on the skin for 5 to 10 minutes to act as a mask, before removing as described.

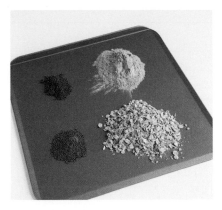

Step 1
Preheat the oven to 100°C (210°F). Place the clay, oats, lime powder and matcha powder on a baking tray (cookie sheet) and transfer to the oven for 30 minutes. Remove from the oven and allow to cool.

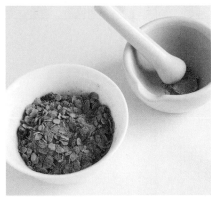

Step 2
Transfer the powder mix to a bowl. Crush the vitamin C tablet and add to the powder mix, then blitz the mixture in a coffee grinder until it has a very fine consistency.

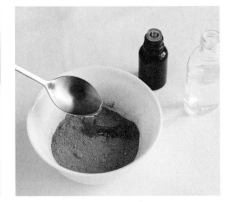

Step 3
Return the powder to the bowl and fold in the Sucragel and the lemon essential oil. Return the mixture to the coffee grinder and blitz again to ensure the ingredients are thoroughly mixed.

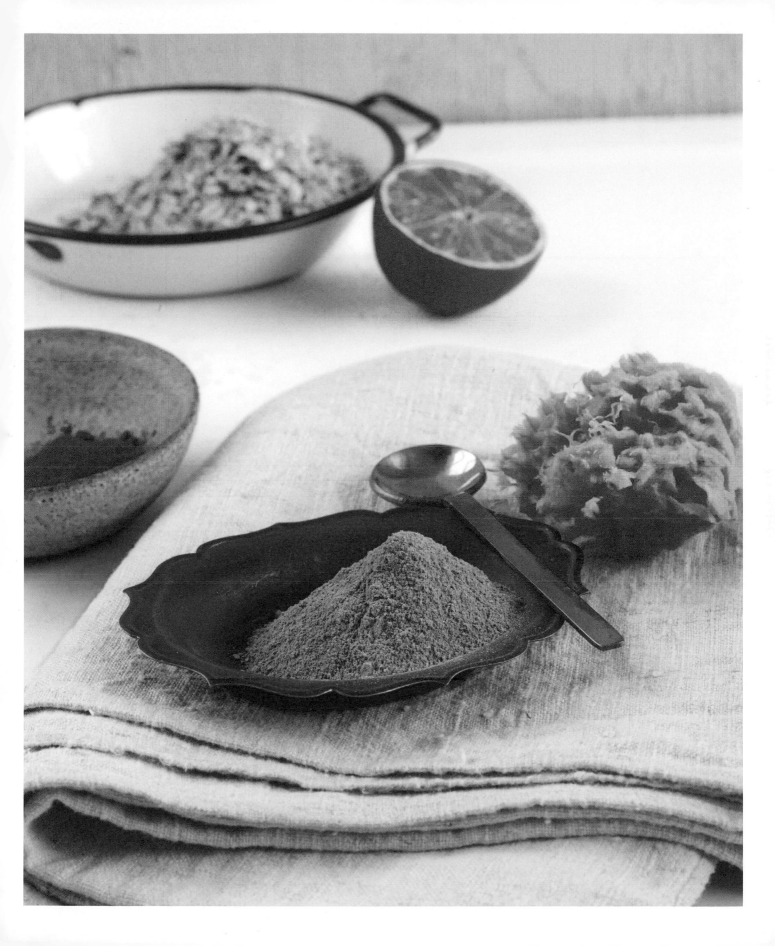

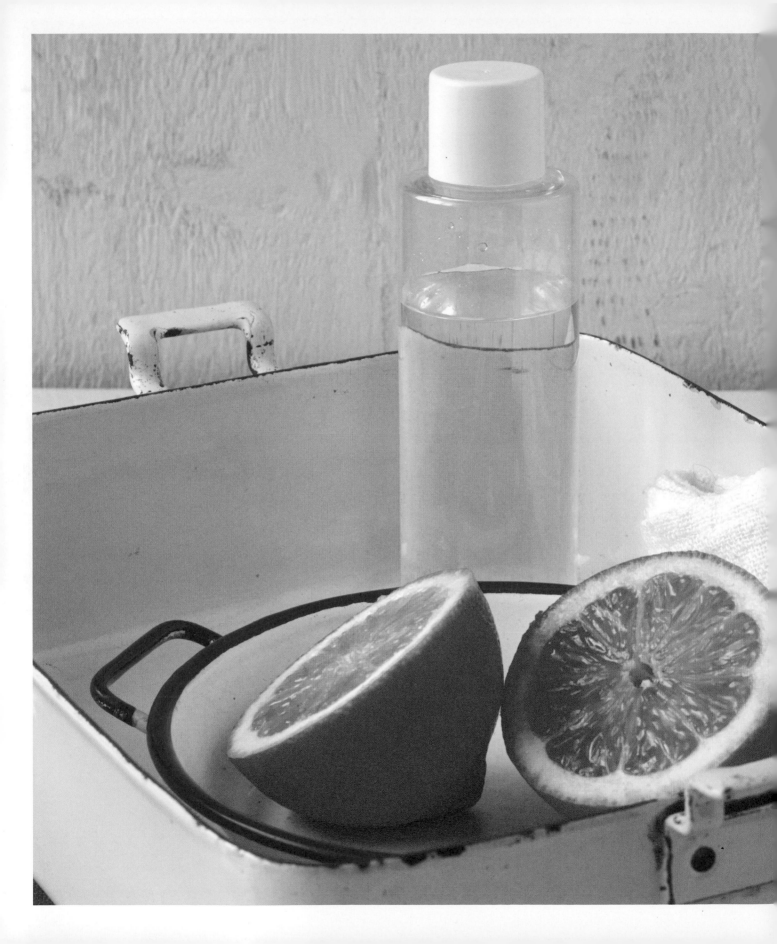

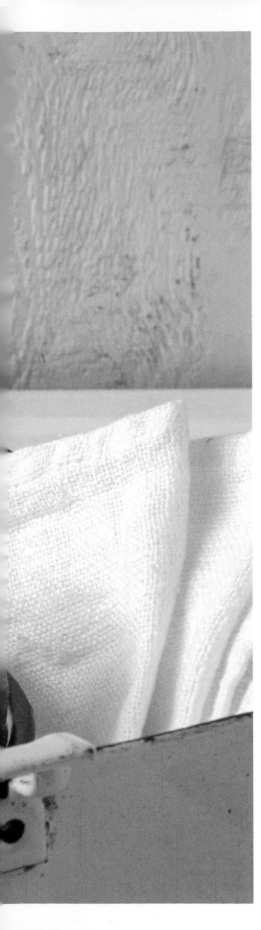

Micellar Cleansing Water

This light, fresh cleansing water removes all traces of make-up effectively and quickly, leaving your skin clean, refreshed and ready for a facial. It can also be used as a Hot Cloth Facial Cleanser (see page 54 for instructions); follow this with a facial spritz (see page 40) to refresh the skin before applying day creams, night creams or serums. The combination of zesty lemon essential oil and orangeflower water makes this the perfect summer weather cleansing solution – and as no added water is required, it's perfect for use on your travels.

Makes approx. 100ml (3½fl oz)

INGREDIENTS	SPECIAL EQUIPMENT
10 drops lemon essential oil	heatproof jug
2.5ml (½ tsp) Plantacare 818	metal saucepan or bain marie
94ml (3fl oz) orangeflower water	sterilized bottle with cap
1.5ml (⅓ tsp) glycerine	
40 drops grapefruit seed	*SAFE STORAGE*
extract	*Store in a cool, dry place, away from sunlight. Keeps for up to 3 months.*

Step 1
To begin, premix the lemon essential oil with the Plantacare 818 in a small dish or jug and set aside.

Step 2
Measure the orangeflower water and glycerine into a heatproof jug. Place the jug in a pan of simmering water or bain marie and heat to 80°C (176°F); you will need to use a thermometer. Maintain this heat for 30 minutes. To avoid excess evaporation, cover the jug with cling film (plastic wrap).

Step 3
Remove the jug from the heat and add the premix, ensuring it is thoroughly combined with the water and glycerine. Allow the liquid to cool to 30–40°C (86–104°F), then add the grapefruit seed extract and stir to mix well. Pour into a sterilized bottle with cap.

HOW TO APPLY
Simply apply to a cotton wool pad and wipe away make-up and the stresses of the day.

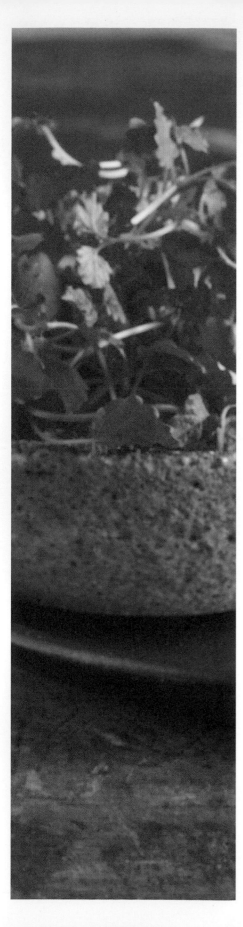

Melissa and Bergamot Facial Spritz

After a hot cloth cleansing treatment (see page 54), spritz this cooling citrus toner on to the face to refresh and revive the skin. Follow with your choice of moisturizer or facial oil for the ultimate facial treatment.

   As an alternative, why not try a rosewater facial spritz to restore and balance the skin. Follow the instructions in steps 1 and 2 below, using rose water in place of the melissa water, and geranium essential oil in place of the bergamot essential oil. All other ingredients remain the same.

Makes approx. 100ml (3½fl oz)

INGREDIENTS
86ml (3fl oz) melissa water
3ml (½ tsp) glycerine
10ml (2 tsp) witch hazel
2 drops bergamot essential oil
40 drops grapefruit seed extract

SPECIAL EQUIPMENT
heatproof jug
saucepan
thermometer
bottle with spray pump

SAFE STORAGE
Store in a cool, dry place, away from sunlight. Keeps for up to 3 months.

Step 1
Measure the melissa water, glycerine and witch hazel into a heatproof jug. Place the jug in a pan of simmering water and heat to 70–80°C (158–176°F); you will need to use a thermometer. Maintain this heat for 30 minutes. To avoid excess evaporation, cover the jug with cling film (plastic wrap).

Step 2
Remove from the heat and allow to cool to 30–40°C (86–104°F). Add the bergamot essential oil and the grapefruit seed extract, pour into the bottle, replace the spray pump and shake to combine.

HOW TO APPLY
Simply spritz on to the face to refresh and revive the skin.

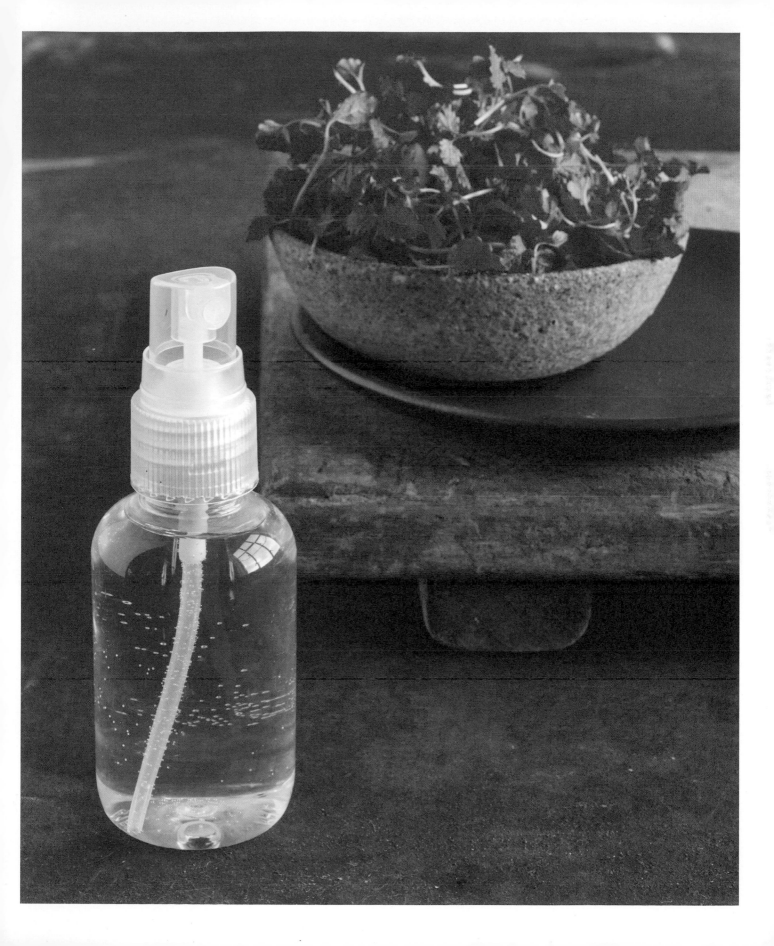

Cooling Cucumber, Matcha and Lime Face Mask

This mask can be made with ingredients that you may already have in your kitchen, and if you use the matcha powder it will have the most amazing, bright green colour. It is a truly zingy, refreshing mask, ideal for a hot, sticky day when its cooling effect can be best appreciated.

Makes approx. 380ml (⅔ pint)

INGREDIENTS
1 green tea bag or 5g (1 tsp) matcha green tea powder (or follow packet instructions)
75g (2½oz) cucumber
2.5g (½ tsp) vegetable gelatine powder, such as Vegeset (or follow packet instructions)
20 drops lime essential oil

SPECIAL EQUIPMENT
blender
small saucepan

SAFE STORAGE
This is a fresh recipe so it should ideally be used straight away. It can be stored in the fridge for up to 2 days, after which it should be discarded.

HOW TO APPLY
Spread the cooling mask over the face and neck and relax while the antioxidant, anti-ageing green tea and cooling, soothing cucumber get to work. Leave for 5 to 10 minutes before removing with warm water and a muslin cloth.

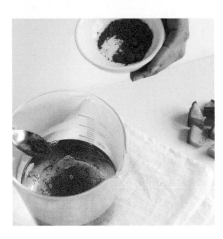

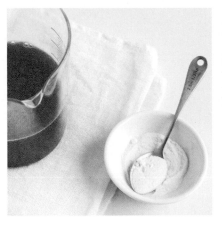

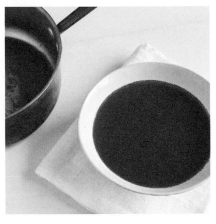

Step 1
Pour 300ml (½ pint) hot (not boiling) water on to the green tea bag or matcha green tea powder in a mug or jug (follow the packet instructions for the correct dosage of powder to water). If using the powder, stir to combine – the liquid will be a bright green colour – then leave to cool slightly. Alternatively, leave the tea bag to infuse for 10 minutes.

Step 2
Chop slices of cucumber and place in a blender with the green tea liquid. Whizz until the cucumber is fully blitzed, then leave to cool completely. Check the amount of liquid and measure out the correct quantity of gelatine powder according to the packet instructions (typically 1 tsp per 600ml/1 pint). Add the gelatine to the liquid and stir to combine.

Step 3
Place the mixture in a pan over a low heat, stirring all the time. Once it has reached boiling point, remove the pan from the heat and allow to cool to around 40°C (104°F). Add the lime essential oil to give a citrus scent: for 300ml (½ pint) use 20 drops (or 10 drops in 150ml/¼ pint). Pour into a bowl and allow to cool before placing in the fridge to set.

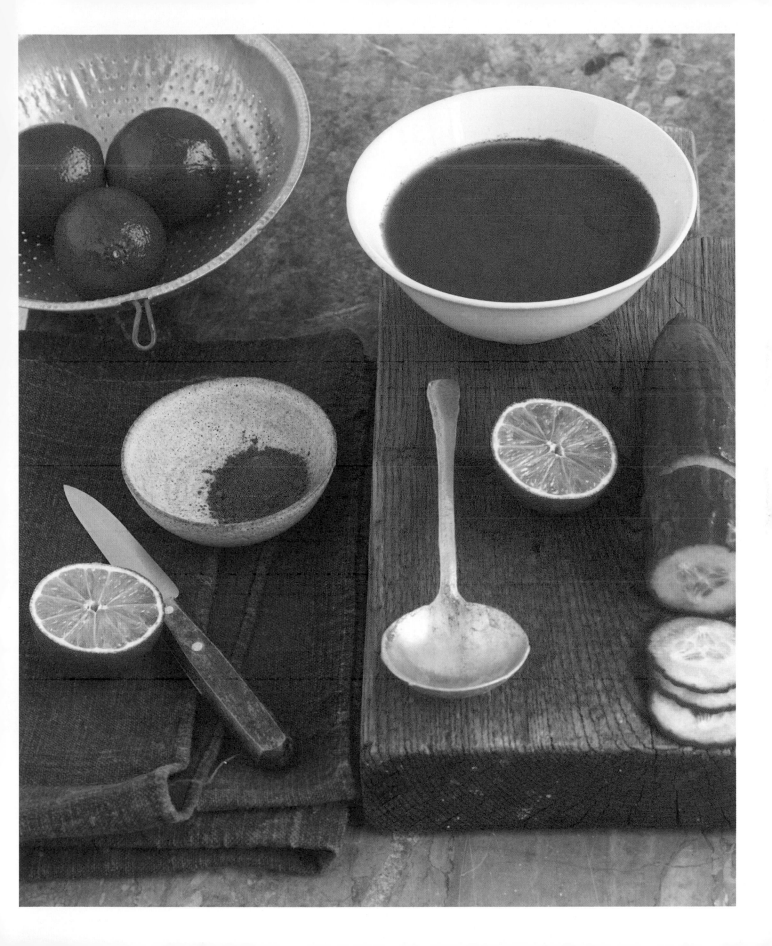

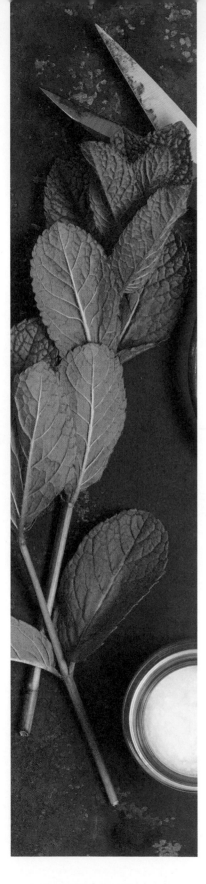

Mint Lip Scrub

When the weather is wintry, our lips feel the full harsh effect of chilling winds and temperatures and need a bit of tender loving care to keep them in good condition. Try this nourishing balm to restore and moisturize parched lips, while gently exfoliating with grains of stevia – an intensely sweet, natural alternative to sugar – leaving a smooth finish. The mint also gives the scrub a lovely taste. This recipe benefits from being made in small amounts and used quickly, as the stevia powder can soften over time, making the exfoliation less effective. The recipe is very simple, so it's easy to whip up another batch when the previous one is finished.

Makes approx. 40g (1½oz)

INGREDIENTS
23g (¾oz) unrefined coconut oil
3g (½ tsp) beeswax
10g (2 tsp) shea butter
4g (1 tsp) stevia
4 drops peppermint essential oil

SPECIAL EQUIPMENT
heatproof jug
metal saucepan

SAFE STORAGE
Store in a cool, dry place, away from sunlight. Keeps for up to 1 month.

Step 1
Weigh the coconut oil, beeswax and shea butter into a heatproof jug. Place the jug in a pan of boiling water and heat until the beeswax is completely molten.

Step 2
When fully melted, remove the jug from the pan, add the stevia, allow the mix to cool slightly, then add the peppermint oil. Stir to combine.

Step 3
Pour or spoon the mixture into the containers just as it is beginning to set, to ensure that the stevia is evenly dispersed and doesn't sink to the base.

HOW TO APPLY
Apply a small amount to the lips, working in the scrub with the fingertips, or by pressing the lips together.

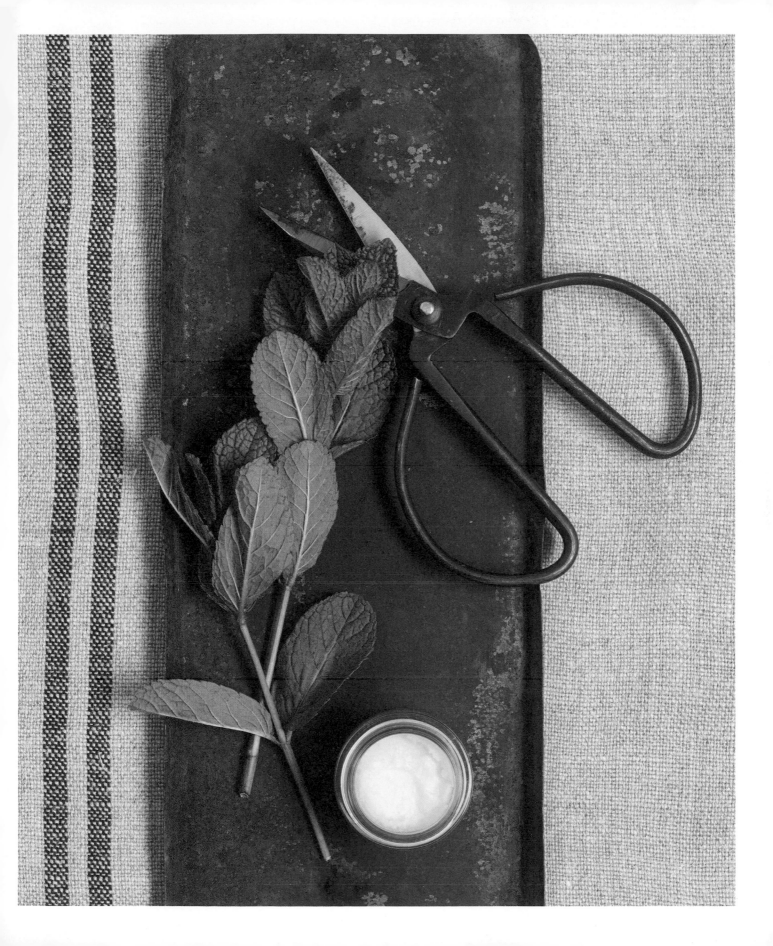

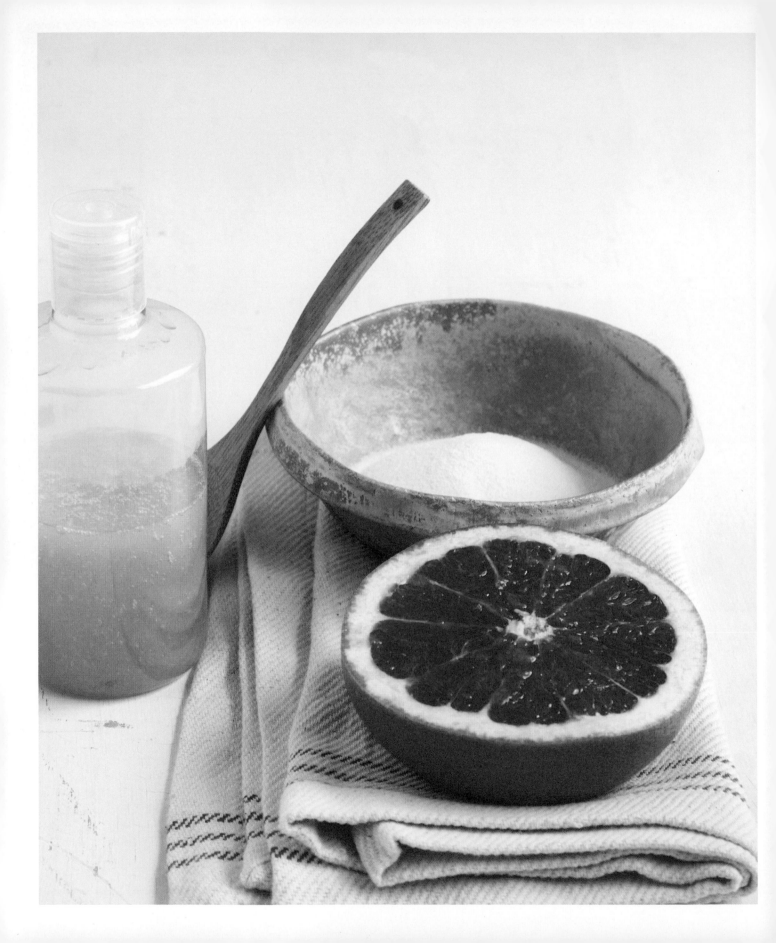

Uplifting Grapefruit and Orange Body Wash

A refreshing, uplifting citrus body wash using mild, natural foaming agents which cleanse and soften the skin, and help bring you to life in the mornings! The wash can also double up as an exfoliating shower treatment – simply mix a small amount of exfoliating powder (there are many options to choose from, but we prefer to use bamboo powder) into the wash in the palm of the hand and apply to the body, paying particular attention to areas of dry skin.

Makes approx. 100ml (3½fl oz)

INGREDIENTS
5ml (1 tsp) glycerine
2g (½ tsp) cellulose gum
40ml (2¾ tbsp) Plantapon LGC
5ml (1 tsp) Lamesoft PO65
46ml (3 tbsp) orangeflower
 water
10 drops grapefruit essential oil
10 drops sweet orange
 essential oil
40 drops grapefruit seed extract

SPECIAL EQUIPMENT
heatproof jug
thermometer
metal saucepan
bottle with cap or lotion pump

SAFE STORAGE
Store in a cool, dry place, away from sunlight. Keeps for up to 3 months.

HOW TO APPLY
The wash is suitable for the hands and all-over body use.

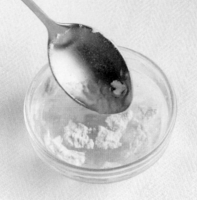

Step 1
Pour the glycerine into a small dish or beaker and add the cellulose gum. Stir to combine until smooth and lump-free, and set aside.

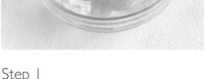

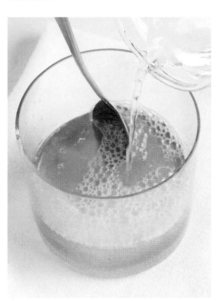

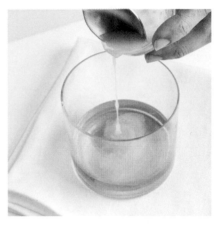

Step 2
Combine the Plantapon LGC and Lamesoft PO65 in a jug or beaker. Add the premix (see Step 1) and stir until the mixture is uniform.

Step 3
Pour the orangeflower water into a heatproof jug. Place the jug in a pan of simmering water and heat to 70–80°C (158–176°F); you will need to use a thermometer. Maintain this heat for 30 minutes. To avoid excess evaporation, cover the jug with cling film (plastic wrap). Leave to cool, then add the orangeflower water to the Plantapon, cellulose gum, glycerine and Lamesoft mix, stirring slowly to avoid adding air and causing foam. Add the essential oils and grapefruit seed extract, and pour into a clean, sterilized bottle; a lotion pump does make application easier.

Refreshing Citrus Fragrance

This zesty perfume is based on traditional, natural citrus-based scents. On a hot summer's day this is the perfect pick-me-up, so carry some with you in a small spray bottle for instant refreshment. The formulation contains all-natural essential oils, so make sure you spray liberally and often for maximum benefit and effect.

Makes approx. 50ml (1½fl oz)

INGREDIENTS

42ml (2¾ tbsp) formulators' alcohol (100%)
15 drops bergamot essential oil
12 drops lemon essential oil
6 drops mandarin essential oil
3 drops rosemary essential oil
5 drops petitgrain essential oil
3 drops benzoin essential oil
3 drops labdanum essential oil
3 drops marjoram essential oil
5.5ml (1 tsp) orangeflower water

SPECIAL EQUIPMENT

optional: cling film (plastic wrap)
optional: glass bottle with lid (for storage)
fine coffee filter paper
glass perfume bottle (for the dressing table) or plastic spray bottle with cap (for on-the-go)

SAFE STORAGE

Store in a cool, dry place away from sunlight. Keeps for up to 12 months.

HOW TO APPLY

Splash or spritz the fragrance on to pulse points as often as desired. The fragrance is very light and fresh and can therefore be used generously, especially in hot weather.

Tip!

The recipe makes a 5% perfume solution based on 1 drop = 0.05ml.

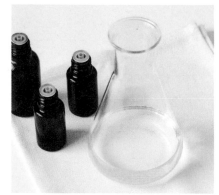

Step 1

Measure the alcohol into a glass measuring jug. Add the drops of essential oils, followed by the orangeflower water and stir to mix thoroughly.

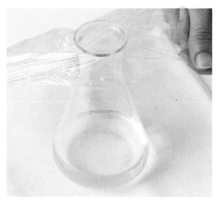

Step 2

Cover the jug with cling film (plastic wrap), or ideally transfer the mixture to a glass bottle with a tightly fitting lid, and leave in a cool place to mature for 5–7 days to allow the fragrance to blend with the alcohol.

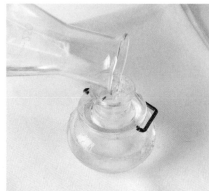

Step 3

Place the jug or bottle in the fridge overnight to bring down any sediment. Pass the fragrance through a fine coffee filter paper, then pour the fragrance into the glass or spray bottle and attach the cap.

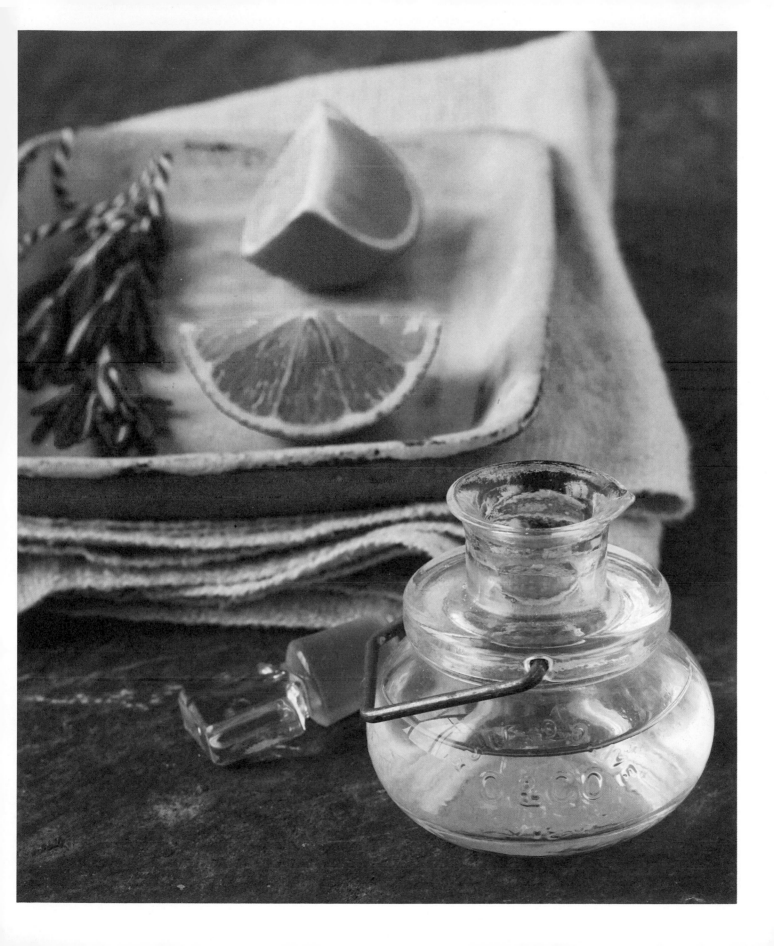

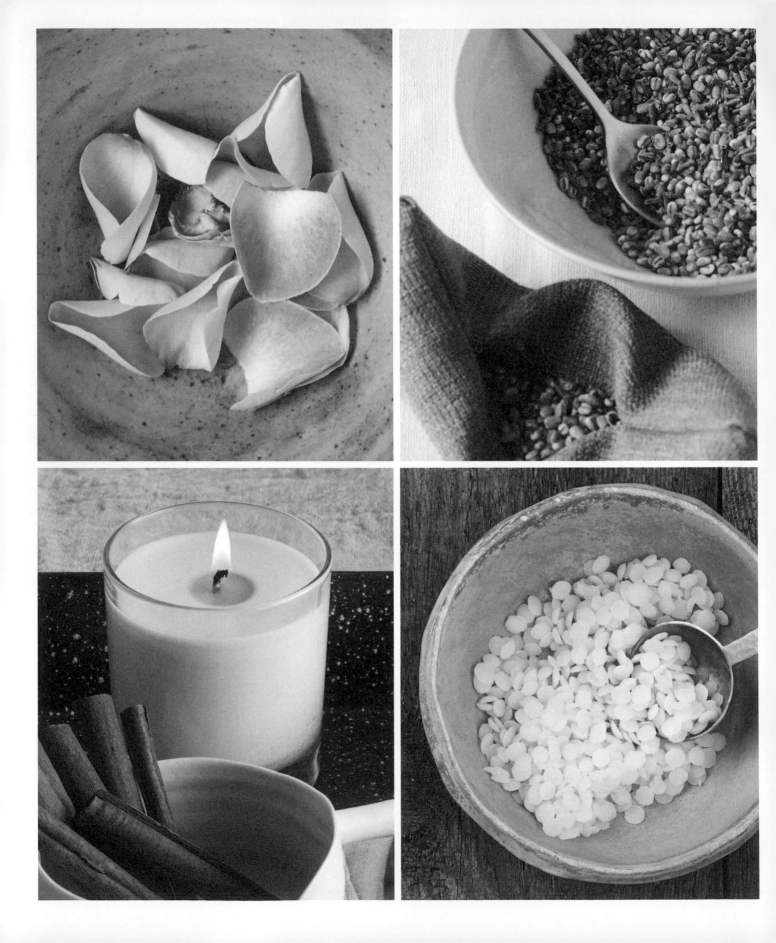

Warming, Relaxing, Soothing

WARMING EXOTIC SPICES, WOODS AND RESINS

SUCH AS GINGER, CINNAMON, SANDALWOOD

AND FRANKINCENSE ARE BLENDED WITH

INDULGENT PLANT TREATMENT OILS TO CREATE

COMFORTING PREPARATIONS TO SOOTHE AND

RELAX A TIRED BODY AND MIND.

Sauna Face Mask with Frankincense and Cypress

This mask has an amazing ability to heat when it comes into contact with the skin. As such it makes a wonderfully warming and soothing winter skin treatment. You will need to allow some time for the ingredients to be heated prior to making the mask, so why not get everything ready, then run a bath or fix a foot spa while you wait.

Makes approx. 100g (3½oz)

INGREDIENTS
10g (2 tsp) kaolin (or a little extra if the mix is too runny)
25g (¾oz) Epsom salts
60ml (2fl oz) glycerine
10 drops frankincense essential oil
10 drops cypress essential oil

SPECIAL EQUIPMENT
baking tray (cookie sheet)

SAFE STORAGE
Ideally, the mask should be used immediately for best effect. Alternatively, it can be stored in an airtight jar in the fridge for 2 days, after which time the warming effect may diminish as the mask absorbs moisture from the surrounding air. Try reheating the mask gently in a 100°C (210°F) oven for about 20 minutes to regenerate the warming properties.

Step 1
Preheat the oven to 100°C (210°F). Place the kaolin and Epsom salts on a baking tray (cookie sheet) and put in the oven for 30 minutes to sterilize the kaolin and desiccate the Epsom salts, which is important for the efficacy of the mask. (The warmth of the mask is generated from the reaction of the Epsom salts regaining moisture from the dampness of the skin, hence the importance of this step.) Remove from the oven and allow to cool.

Step 2
Place the dry ingredients in a clean, dry bowl or glass jug. Add the glycerine and the essential oils and mix thoroughly.

HOW TO APPLY
Ensure the skin is damp before applying the mask to the face and neck, avoiding the eye area. Massage into the skin and leave on for 5 to 10 minutes, then rinse the face with warm water or hot cloths to remove all traces of the mask.

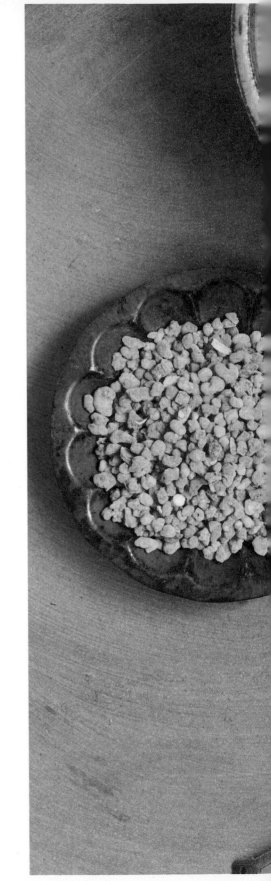

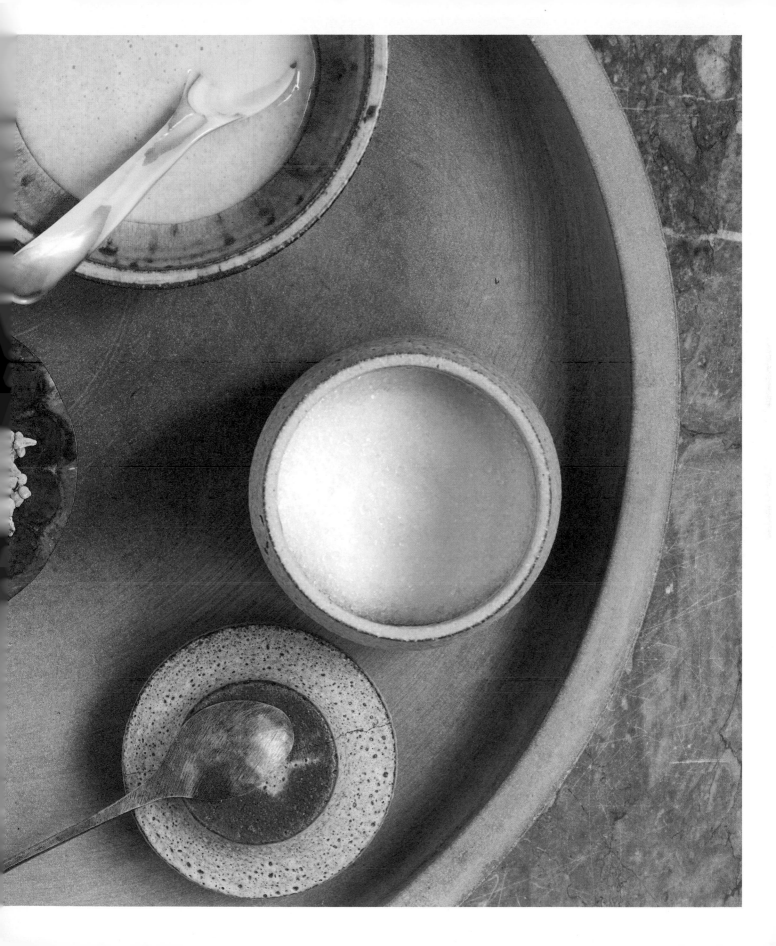

Hot Cloth Facial Cleansers

Hot cloth cleansing is truly reminiscent of luxury spas: just imagine the sheer relaxation of experiencing a facial using muslin cloths at just the right temperature to take all that stress away, while at the same time giving an amazing, deep cleansing treatment. We also love them when they are handed out in a restaurant at the end of a great meal, sometimes using them on our faces as well as our hands because it just feels fabulous. If you love this kind of treatment, then why not try it as part of a pampering skincare treat when you're at home. Choose the cleansing water recipe that best suits your skin (see pages 39 and 56–7). Each one contains both beneficial aromatic essential oils and extracts as well as the Plantacare ingredients that will help to cleanse the skin.

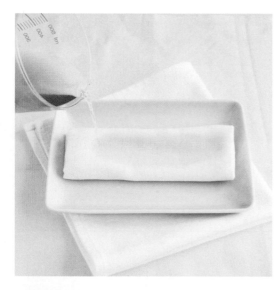

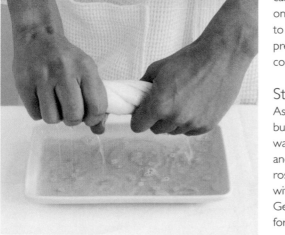

INSTRUCTIONS FOR USE

If you are using the hot cloth cleansers on your face, it is very important to remove all make-up first using a good cleanser such as our Calming Facial Cleansing Balm (see page 88).

Step 1

Choose a comfortable place in which to relax and experience your treatment. Place a muslin facecloth in a microwaveable dish and pour sufficient cleansing water on to the cloth so that it is damp and has absorbed the solution. Cover and place in the microwave for 1 minute. Check that the temperature of the cloth is just right: it must be really warm, but not too hot. Repeat the heating if the cloth is not warm enough and always check carefully before using.

Step 2

Remove the cloth from the dish and wring out the excess water, so that the cloth is not dripping wet. Lay it delicately over your face, so the steam can open up your pores and allow the cleanser and essential oils to work on your skin. Relax and enjoy the experience, allowing the warming cloth to soothe your skin. You may find that holding the warm cloth and gently pressing around the temples and the sides of your nose will help to ease any congestion and associated tension.

Step 3

As the skin has been pre-cleansed there should be no need to rinse the cloth, but you may wish to repeat the treatment with a second cloth to prolong the warming, beneficial action. Follow the hot cloth treatment with our Melissa and Bergamot Facial Spritz (see page 40) for a refreshing pick me up, or the rosewater variation (see page 40) for a restorative, balancing treatment. Finish with your chosen moisturizer, such as the Facial Serum with Pomegranate and Geranium (see page 76), or the Regenerating Rose Facial Oil (see page 78) for a richer, night-time treatment.

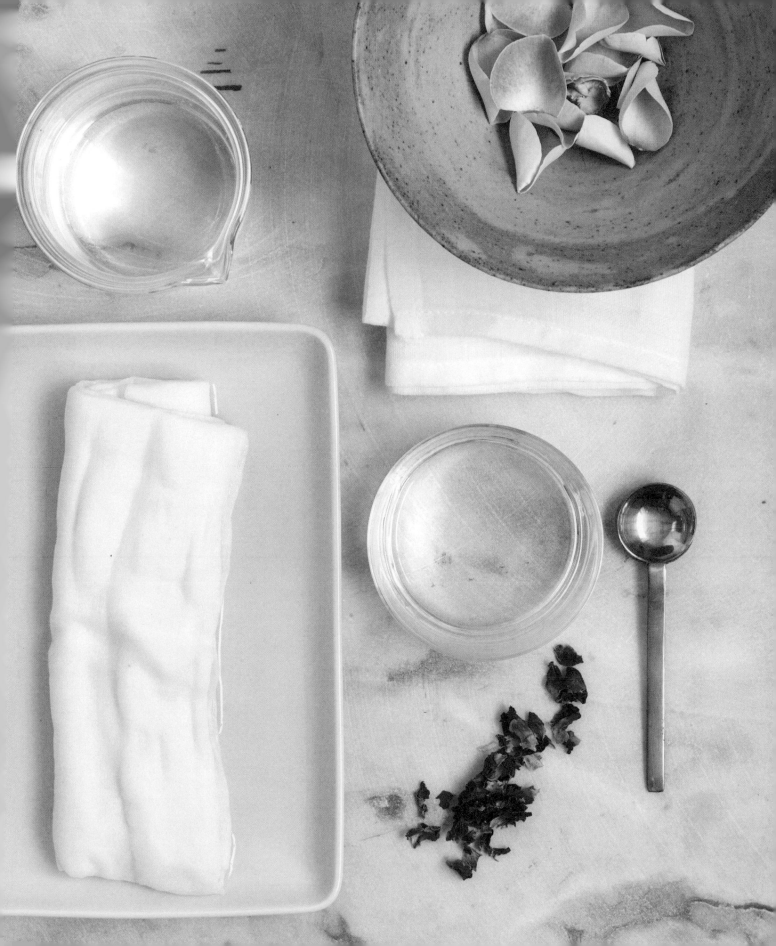

Detoxifying Seaweed Cleansing Water

You don't need to live by the sea and have access to fresh seaweed to make this reviving cleansing water; simply use dried seaweed, which can be purchased online (see Directory of Suppliers, page 142), and follow the packet instructions to create the infusion. The resulting water is a beautiful pale green, as relaxing to look at as it is to use.

Makes approx. 100ml (3½fl oz)

INGREDIENTS
93ml (3¼fl oz) seaweed
  infusion (from dried seaweed
  and water, see Step 1)
2.5ml (½ tsp) Plantacare 818
1.5ml (⅓ tsp) glycerine
5 drops fennel essential oil
5 drops thyme essential oil
40 drops grapefruit seed
  extract

SPECIAL EQUIPMENT
metal sieve
heatproof jug
sterilized bottle with cap

SAFE STORAGE
Store in a cool, dry place, away from sunlight. Keeps for up to 3 months.

HOW TO APPLY
Follow the instructions on page 54 for how to use the hot cloth facial treatments to best effect.

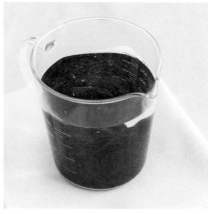

Step 1
Combine the dried seaweed with water, according to the packet instructions, and leave to infuse.

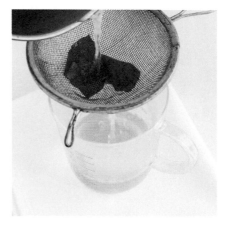

Step 2
Measure out the amount required for the recipe, using a metal sieve to filter out the dried seaweed.

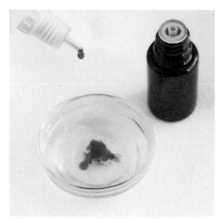

Step 3
In a small dish, premix the Plantacare 818 with the glycerine and essential oils, then add the grapefruit seed extract.

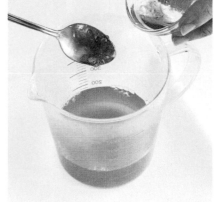

Step 4
Add this mixture to the seaweed infusion and stir to combine completely. Pour into a sterilized bottle with a cap.

Regenerating Rose Cleansing Water

This gentle, clear cleansing water has the power to cleanse the skin effectively and quickly.

Makes approx. 100ml (3½fl oz)

INGREDIENTS
93ml (3¼fl oz) rose water
2.5ml (½ tsp) Plantacare 818
1.5ml (⅓ tsp) glycerine
40 drops grapefruit seed extract

SPECIAL EQUIPMENT
heatproof jug
metal saucepan or bain marie
thermometer
sterilized bottle and cap

Measure the rose water, Plantacare 818 and glycerine into a heatproof jug and stir to combine. Place the jug in a pan of simmering water or bain marie and heat to 80°C (176°F); you will need to use a thermometer. Maintain this heat for 30 minutes. To avoid excess evaporation, cover the jug with cling film (plastic wrap).

Remove from the heat and allow the liquid to cool to 30–40°C (86–104°F), then add the grapefruit seed extract and mix well. Pour into a sterilized bottle with cap.

SAFE STORAGE
Store in a cool, dry place, away from sunlight. Keeps for up to 3 months.

HOW TO APPLY
Follow the instructions on page 54 for how to use the hot cloth facial treatments to best effect.

Restful Lavender Cleansing Water

This variation on the Regenerating Rose Cleansing Water uses lavender water as a base.

Makes approx. 100ml (3½fl oz)

INGREDIENTS
93ml (3¼fl oz) lavender water
2.5ml (½ tsp) Plantacare 818
1.5ml (⅓ tsp) glycerine
40 drops grapefruit seed extract

SPECIAL EQUIPMENT
heatproof jug
metal saucepan or bain marie
thermometer
sterilized bottle with cap

Measure the lavender water, Plantacare 818 and glycerine into a heatproof jug and stir to combine. Place the jug in a pan of simmering water or bain marie and heat to 80°C (176°F); you will need to use a thermometer. Maintain this heat for 30 minutes. To avoid excess evaporation, cover the jug with cling film (plastic wrap).

Remove from the heat and allow the liquid to cool to 30–40°C (86–104°F), then add the grapefruit seed extract and mix well. Pour into a sterilized bottle with cap.

SAFE STORAGE
Store in a cool, dry place, away from sunlight. Keeps for up to 3 months.

HOW TO APPLY
Follow the instructions on page 54 for how to use the hot cloth facial treatments to best effect.

Warming, Sensual Body Massage Oil

This deliciously scented body massage oil contains warming ginger blended with sensual frankincense and ylang ylang and balanced by calming rose geranium. The nourishing oil blend sinks naturally into the skin, but has just the right amount of play to make a perfect massage oil. Although the recipe has a long list of ingredients, you will find it very quick and simple to make, with no heating or special mixing, so if you find that you have used up a batch, you can quickly make another.

Makes approx. 100ml (3½fl oz)

INGREDIENTS
30ml (2 tbsp) rapeseed oil
5ml (1 tsp) evening primrose oil
40ml (2¾ tbsp) sweet almond oil
5ml (1 tsp) rosehip oil
10ml (2 tsp) grapeseed oil
9ml (2¾ tsp) olive oil
5 drops rose geranium essential oil
5 drops ginger essential oil
5 drops frankincense essential oil
5 drops ylang ylang essential oil

SPECIAL EQUIPMENT
sterilized bottle and cap

SAFE STORAGE
Store in a cool, dry place, away from sunlight. Keeps for up to 6 months.

Step 1
Measure the ingredients into a beaker or jug in the exact order shown above. Stir thoroughly to mix the vegetal oils and the essential oils together, then pour into the sterilized bottle and seal.

Massage has an amazing ability to release tension and soothe both body and mind; the action of massage releases endorphins, which improve our sense of well-being. The techniques on the opposite page can be useful in providing both self-massage and simple treatments for a partner.

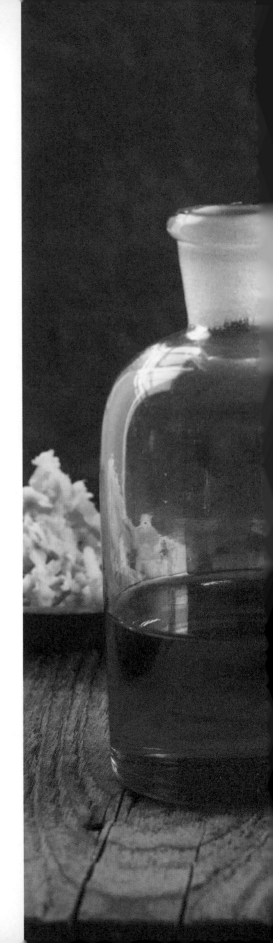

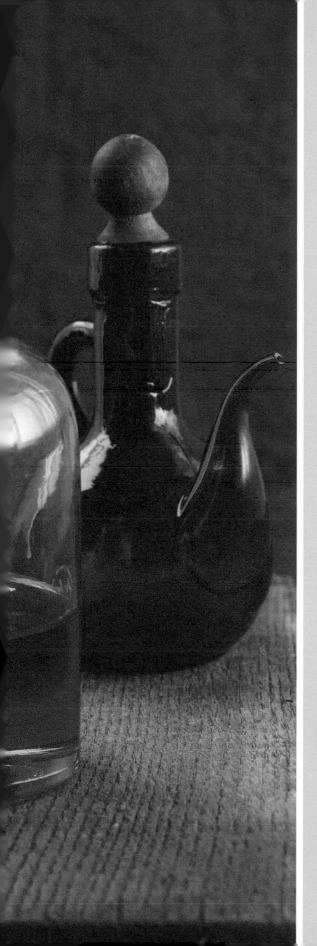

Massage Techniques

SELF-MASSAGE

Practise slow, deep abdominal breathing, often known as yoga breathing. Close your eyes and stroke your fingers from the bridge of your nose over the eyebrows to the temples. Then apply gentle pressure to the temples and below the cheekbones, which will help to clear blocked sinuses and ease tension. With your hands on the sides of your head, place your thumbs into the indentations at the base of the skull and hold for 5 to 10 seconds, then release.

To ease tension in the neck and shoulders, place your left hand on your right shoulder and squeeze the flesh between your palm and fingers. Hold for a few seconds and release. Applying gentle pressure, use the fingertips to massage the side of the neck and top of the shoulder, working into any knots. Stroke the area using downward movements, then repeat on the other side.

PARTNER MASSAGE

Check that your partner is not pregnant, or has contra-indications to any specific essential oils you plan to use. Ensure that the room is warm and that your partner is relaxed and comfortable. With your partner lying flat, face down on a bed or thick blanket, place a rolled-up towel under their head to keep the back and neck straight and well supported during the massage. You can also place a rolled-up towel under their feet.

BACK MASSAGE

Place a small amount of the massage oil in your palms and rub the hands together to warm them before you begin. Place your hands on your partner's lower back on either side of the spine. Slowly stroke up the back and over the shoulders, fanning your hands out at the top of the shoulders, then glide your hands lightly down the sides of the body. Repeat 4 or 5 times.

Starting at the base of the spine, use your thumbs to make circular outward pressing movements on either side of the spine. Continue this movement over the upper back and shoulders to the neck, which may feel knotted and tight as it is where many people hold tension. Cup your fingers around the base of the neck and stroke up to the hairline in a continuous movement using gentle pressure with the fingers and thumb. Repeat about 8 times.

Finish the massage with some cat strokes. Using the palms of your hands, stroke alternate hands down your partner's back, from the shoulder to the base of the spine; as one hand comes to the end of a stroke, the other takes over, creating a continuous rhythmic movement. Finally, place your warm hands on your partner's lower back for about a minute, using gentle pressure, then finally circle the hands once and remove them, holding them briefly above your partner who will feel the heat coming from them.

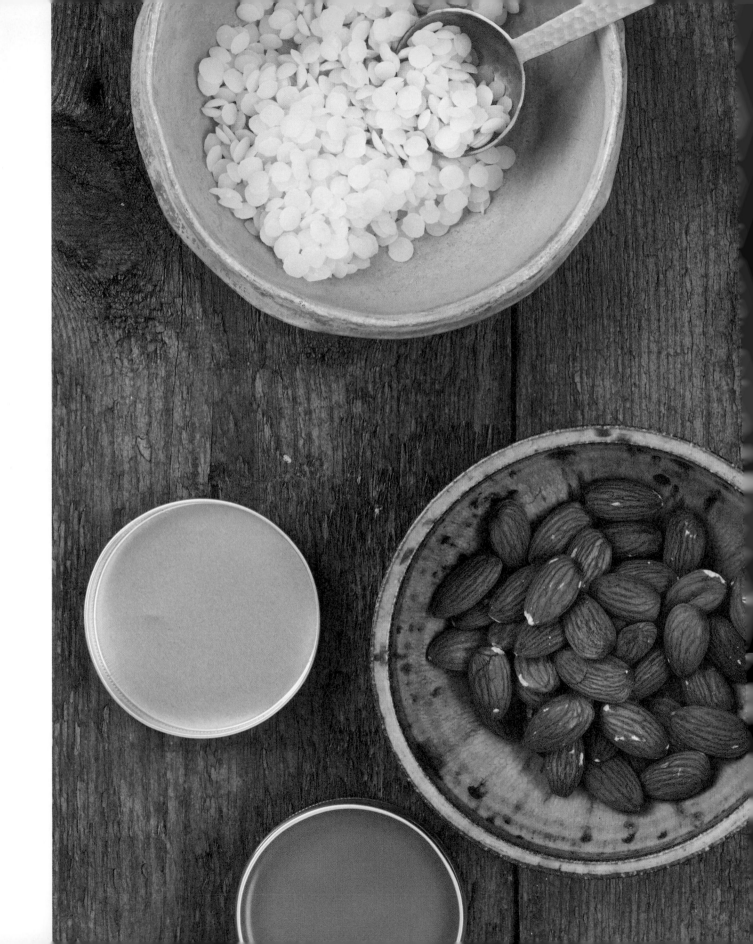

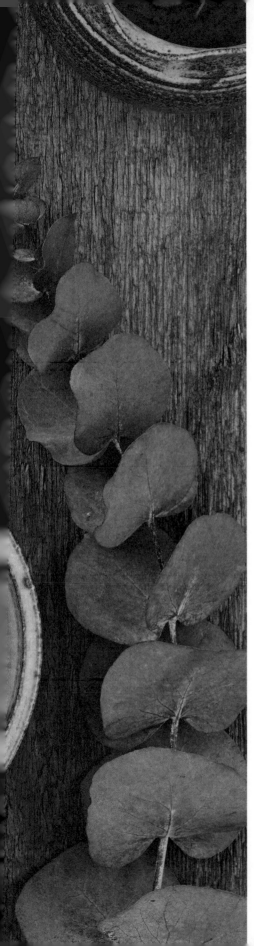

Ginger, Eucalyptus and Cinnamon Muscle Balm

This warming balm is our version of Tiger Balm, but uses moisturizing wheatgerm and sweet almond oil with beeswax as a natural base, and a blend of eucalyptus and spicy essential oils to help soothe tired and aching muscles. If you put the balm into a small jar or mini tin, the recipe becomes easily transportable, so is very handy for use when travelling. It is also ideal for use after sporting activities or a spot of gardening.

Makes approx. 50g (1¾oz)

INGREDIENTS
20ml (1⅓ tbsp) wheatgerm oil
22ml (1½ tbsp) sweet almond oil
5g (1 tsp) beeswax
30 drops eucalyptus essential oil
35 drops cinnamon essential oil
35 drops ginger essential oil

SPECIAL EQUIPMENT
heatproof jug
metal saucepan or bain marie
sterilized glass jars and lids

SAFE STORAGE
Store in a cool, dry place, away from sunlight. Keeps for up to 6 months.

Step 1
Measure the wheatgerm and sweet almond oils and beeswax into a heatproof jug.

Step 2
Place the jug in a pan of simmering water and heat until melted. Remove from the heat and allow to cool until the mixture just begins to show signs of cloudiness.

Step 3
Add the essential oils and stir to ensure they are thoroughly mixed. Pour into a sterilized jar (or 2 smaller jars) with a lid.

HOW TO APPLY
Massage the balm gently into areas of stiffness, such as the back and shoulders, to warm and soothe muscles. Do not use on the face or around the eye area.

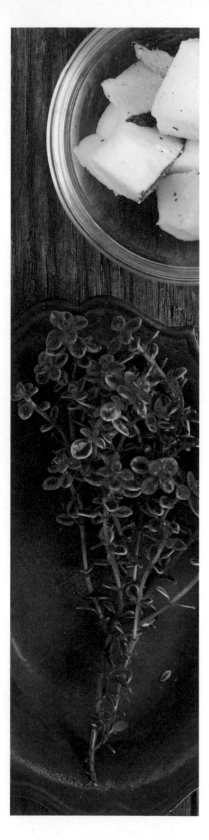

Hot Oil Hair Treatment Mask

This recipe is something of a trip down memory lane for those who remember the hot oil hair treatments of the 1970s and 1980s. As we love old recipes, we thought this one was just about due for a revival using the natural ingredients and oils around today. So get your favourite old vinyl records out and dance around the kitchen with your hair wrapped in a towel, giving it a superb, nourishing treatment at the same time.

Makes approx. 100ml (3½fl oz)

INGREDIENTS
84ml (2¾fl oz) fractionated coconut oil
4ml (¾ tsp) argan oil
3ml (½ tsp) baobab oil
3ml (½ tsp) meadowfoam oil
5ml (1 tsp) Polysorbate 20
3 drops sandalwood essential oil
4 drops thyme essential oil
3 drops rosemary essential oil

SPECIAL EQUIPMENT
glass bottle and cap
heatproof jug

SAFE STORAGE
Store in a cool, dry place, away from sunlight. Keeps for up to 3 months.

Step 1
Place the coconut, argan, baobab and meadowfoam oils into a glass bottle, followed by the Polysorbate 20, and stir to combine thoroughly. Add the essential oils and continue to mix until clear.

Step 2
Place the bottle into a heatproof jug and pour hot (not boiling) water into the jug around the bottle, so that the height of the water is almost at the height of the liquid in the bottle. Leave the bottle in the jug for around 5 minutes, until the oil is warm (not hot) to the touch, then remove from the jug using a tea towel if the bottle is hot.

HOW TO APPLY
Pour a small amount of the warm oil into the palm of the hand. Apply to dry or damp hair, spreading the oil along the hair shaft to coat it. Wrap the hair in a towel and leave for 20 minutes, then shampoo and rinse the hair as normal afterwards.

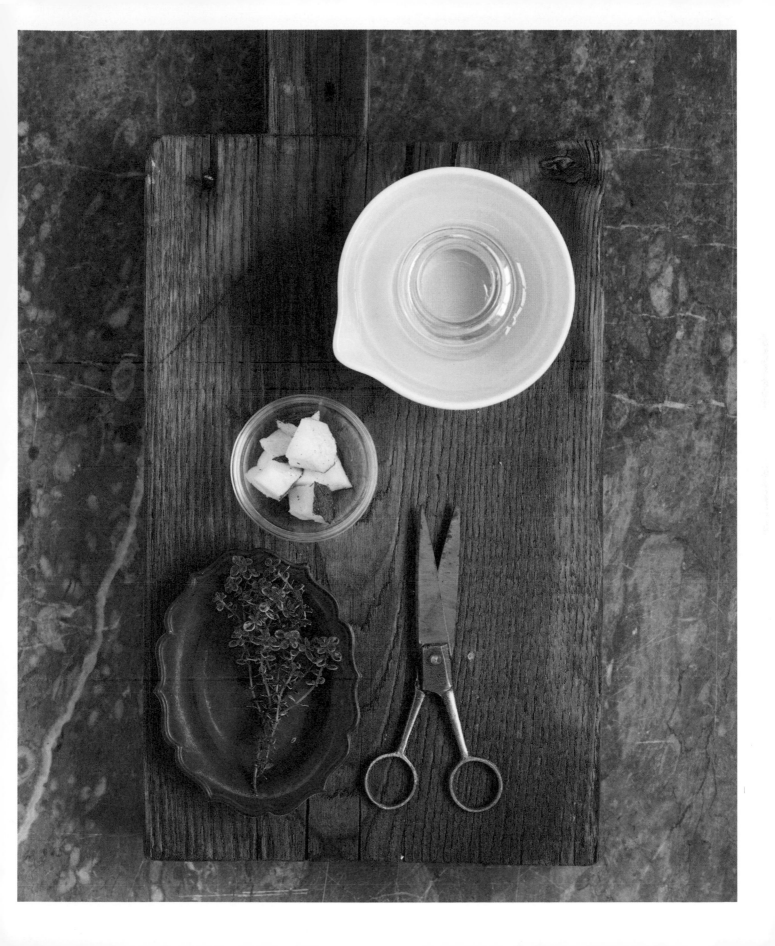

Hot or Cold Soothing Wheat Pack

A wheat pack is so versatile! It can be heated to soothe aching muscles and aid relaxation, or chilled to create a cooling, restful eye mask, which blocks out the light and aids sleep. The addition of fragrant lavender flowers adds to the relaxing qualities. This project is so simple to make from small pieces of fabric and would make a perfect gift.

INGREDIENTS
pearl barley or rice
dried lavender flowers
optional: lavender essential oil

SPECIAL EQUIPMENT
cotton fabric
scissors
pins
sewing machine
cotton sewing thread (to
  match fabric)
iron
needle

SAFE STORAGE
Store in a cool, dry place away from sunlight. Keeps for up to 12 months, but the life of the wheat pack may be reduced by repeated use.

HOW TO APPLY
To create a warming pack, place a glass bowl of water in a microwave, then place the wheat pack alongside. Heat for 1–2 minutes on high, then lay the pack across aching muscles. To use as a cooling mask for tired eyes, place the pack in a plastic bag in the fridge to chill. Remove the bag, lay the pack across the eyes and relax.

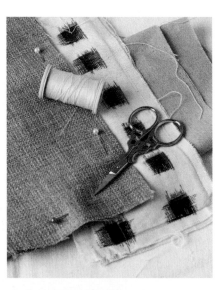

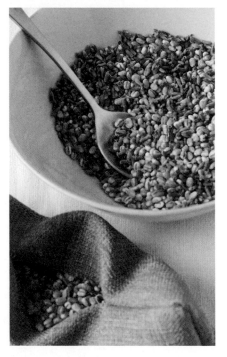

Step 1
Choose the fabric for your wheat pack and fold it in half so you have a double thickness of material. Measure the desired amount of fabric – for an eye mask, use 20 x 9cm (8 x 3.5in); for a warming pack use 50 x 12cm (20.5 x 4.5in) – allowing an extra 1cm (0.5in) all around for a seam. Cut out the 2 rectangles of fabric, then place the 2 pieces together with the right sides facing inwards and the wrong sides facing out. Pin the four sides together, leaving a 2.5cm (1in) gap in the seam for filling. Using a sewing machine, stitch the seams and turn the bag right side out. Press the seams flat with an iron.

Step 2
Estimate the amount of filling required, but remember that the bag should not be completely full as it needs to fold around the body. Pour the pearl barley into a bowl, then add the lavender flowers and mix together well so the flowers are evenly dispersed. Allow around 20% lavender to 80% pearl barley. If the scent seems faint, add a few drops of lavender oil to the mix, but do remember that anything placed on the face doesn't need to be very strong. If you do this, ensure the filling is dry before proceeding. Spoon the lavender and pearl barley into the hole in the pack until it is about three-quarters full. With your needle and thread, slip stitch the open seam to close it.

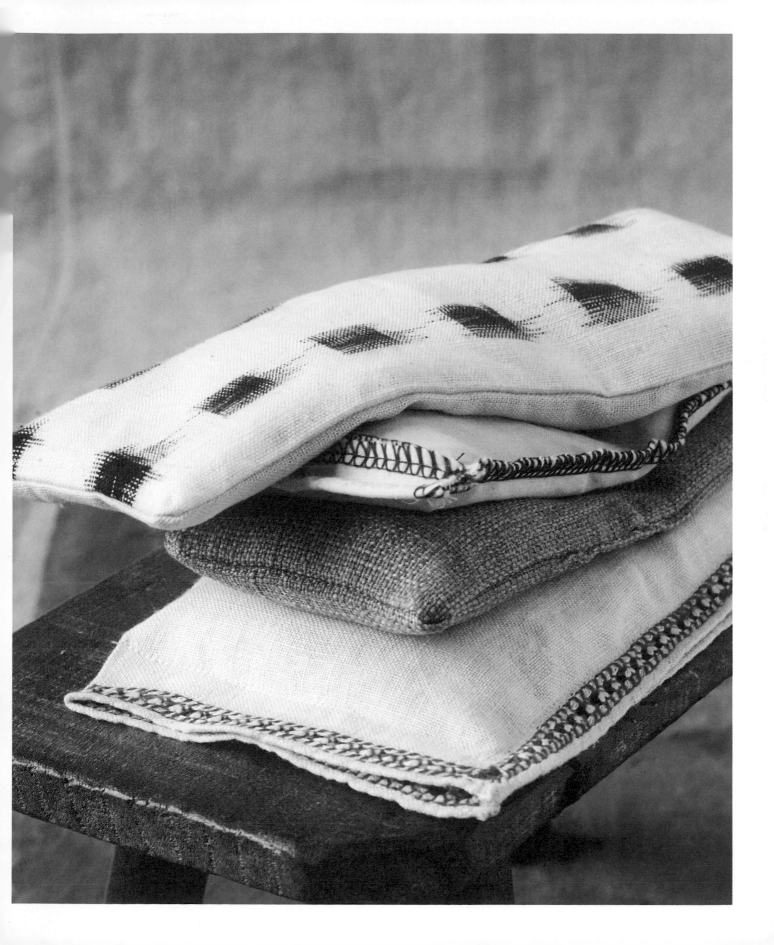

Scented Candles

All good-quality candles are expensive, so why not make your own? You are able to use natural wax rather than paraffin wax, and can tailor the choice of fragrance or essential oils to your mood – creating a candle to lift your spirits or to complement a relaxing spa experience.

The percentage of fragrance or essential oils in the wax blend for your candle should be between 5 and 8 per cent. If using fragrance oils, they must be designed specifically for candles or they may not work as well. Fragrance oils can have a more powerful scent than essential oils, and can also be more affordable, as you do need a relatively large amount of oil, making essential oils an expensive prospect.

You will need:

- Glass or ceramic containers are ideal for scented candles. For a candle with a single wick you could use a standard drinking glass with a diameter of around 8cm, or a smaller votive glass. Larger containers require multiple wicks, which is a more complex undertaking. They also generate a fair amount of heat and can be more of a fire risk, so we prefer to stick to single-wick candles for our spa experience.
- You will need to choose the correct wick size for your candles from a specialist supplier; the wick needs to be appropriate for the wax you have chosen and for the size of your container, so do check with your supplier as they will be able to guide you in the right direction. It's important to set the wick right in the centre and to keep it straight – we use wick stickers on the base of the container to hold the wick in place, and use a wick holder or place wooden skewers around the wick to hold it straight.
- To achieve a good finish when making scented candles, you need to pour the wax in two stages. The first pour is the main pour, to around 2cm below the rim. The second and final top-up ensures there are no dips in the top of the candle and gives a professional finish.

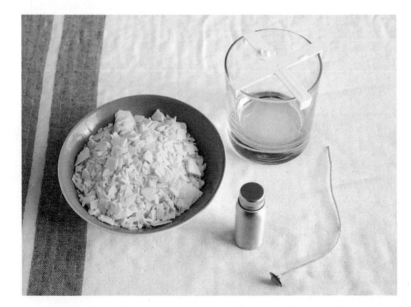

SAFETY

- *Keep candles away from anything that may catch fire – curtains, bedding, furniture etc. Always place them on a stable, heat-resistant surface.*
- *Never burn candles for more than 4 hours at a time.*
- *Extinguish all candles when leaving a room or going to sleep.*
- *Pinch off the end of the wick in between burns; don't cut it. Allow the candle to cool before relighting.*

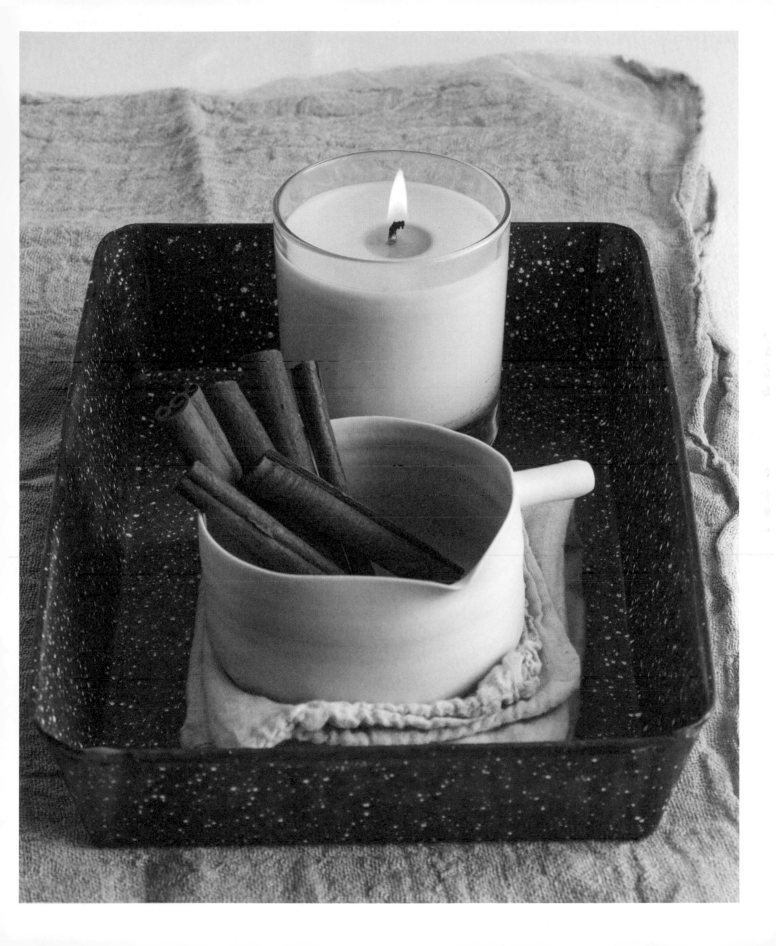

Tips

When pouring the wax, hold a piece of kitchen towel (paper towel) in your other hand to wipe drips from the pourer.

Leftover wax can be melted and reused, if desired. Do not dispose of wax down the sink or drains: it will set and cause a blockage. Pour or scrape any unwanted wax on to paper and place it in the bin.

Clean all tools and equipment with kitchen towel (paper towel) to remove wax before washing with detergent.

PREPARATION

• Cover work area with an old cloth or newspaper to catch any drips or spillages of wax.
• Wear an apron to protect your clothing from wax spillages.
• Make sure your containers are clean and dry.
• Measure the volume of your chosen container with water and weigh out the same amount of wax.
• Calculate the amount of fragrance required, based on the amount of wax you are using (see Materials).
• Cut up the wax into smaller pieces if necessary; this will help the wax to melt evenly.

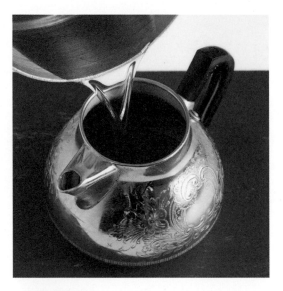

Step 1

Place the wax into the top pan of a bain marie/double boiler and melt. Keep an eye on the water level; do not allow it to boil dry. Once melted, check the temperature of the wax: it should be 60°C (140°F) or just below, but check the supplier's instructions for recommended pouring temperature. Remove from the heat and leave to cool if necessary. Warm the jug or pourer with hot water, and dry the inside before pouring the wax into the warm pourer.

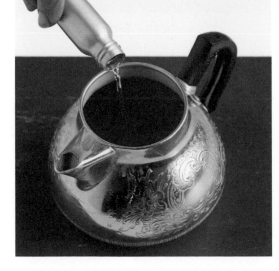

Step 2

Add the fragrance or essential oils to the melted wax in the pourer and stir well with a skewer to disperse fully. It is important to keep the temperature of the wax at or below 60°C (140°F) after adding the fragrance, as higher temperatures change the scent.

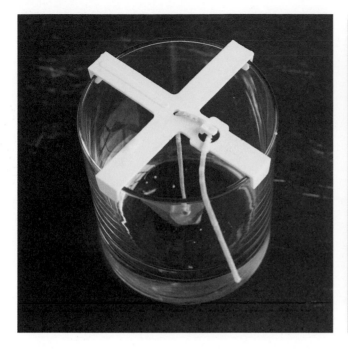

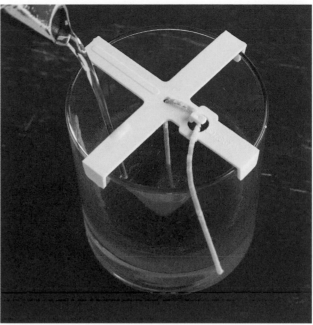

Step 3

Place a wick sticker centrally in the base of each container, then place the wick sustainer on top and secure in place. Check the wick is straight. If necessary, place wooden skewers crosswise around the wick to keep it straight, or ideally use a wick holder designed to fit the size of your container.

Step 4

Before you fill them, ensure that the containers you've chosen have no cracks or flaws. Carefully pour the wax from the pourer into the glass containers, and fill to 2cm below the rim. Keep the remaining wax warm over a low heat.

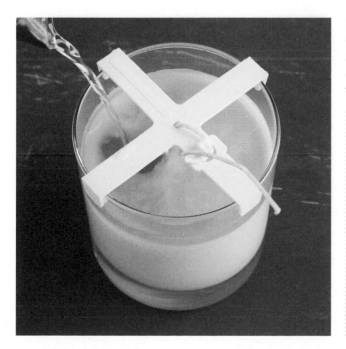

Step 5

Once a thick skin has formed on the wax in the container, after around 10 minutes, depending on the room temperature and candle size, top the container up to 1cm from the rim and leave to set fully.

> ### USING AND STORING CANDLES
>
> *When making candles, ensure that they are fully cold before attempting to light them, and ideally leave them for 2 days before lighting them for the first time.*
>
> *It is important to store candles away from heat and ensure that no dust or debris falls into the candle, as this can cause secondary burning. Candle lids are available which fit many standard-sized containers, helping to keep your candle clean and dust-free when not in use.*

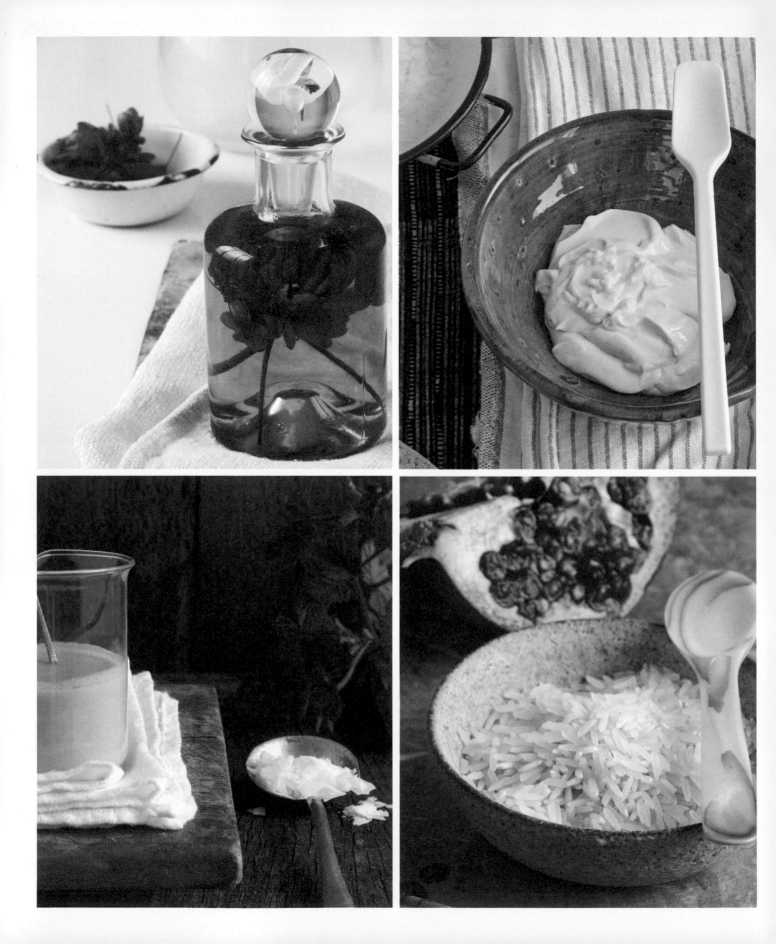

Regenerating, Balancing

PLANTS AND FLOWERS IN THEIR ORIGINAL
FORM ARE USED HERE ALONGSIDE
POWERFUL FLOWER OILS SUCH AS YLANG
YLANG, GERANIUM AND NEROLI, AS WELL
AS PRECIOUS OILS FROM SLEMONGRASS
AND POMEGRANATE, TO CREATE INSPIRING
RESTORATIVE, BALANCING TREATMENTS.

Facial Steam with Floating Flowers

Facial steams help to clear the pores, detoxify the skin and promote circulation. They can also be very relaxing, providing an opportunity to breathe deeply and allow a few moments of calm and meditation. The steam does most of the work, but you can augment its effect by adding some beneficial botanicals to the water.

- Detoxing and Cleansing: fennel, lemon and grapefruit peel, mint and wild pansy
- Relaxing and Soothing: lavender, camomile, marjoram, lime flowers and primrose
- Problem Skin: thyme, rosemary and marigold
- Dry Skin: camomile, rose and geranium (pelargonium leaves)

Makes approx. 100ml (3½fl oz)

INGREDIENTS	SPECIAL EQUIPMENT
your chosen herbs and flowers – try sourcing these from the garden, the hedgerow, or even from your local florist, supermarket or greengrocer	large bowl heatproof mat bath towel

Step 1
Add a small handful of your chosen herbs or flowers to a large bowl and cover with boiling water. Leave to cool slightly.

Step 2
Place a heatproof mat on the table and place the bowl on top. Make sure the bowl is conveniently placed just in front of your face and that you are seated comfortably. Lean over the bowl so that the steam wafts around you. Then place a large bath towel over your head to create a steam tent, ensuring there are no gaps for the steam to escape.

HOW TO APPLY
Breathe deeply and enjoy the scented steam. Take this time to completely clear the mind of any concerns or worries and to be present in the moment. You may wish to use a timer to set the amount of time you think appropriate for the treatment, 5 to 10 minutes is about right.

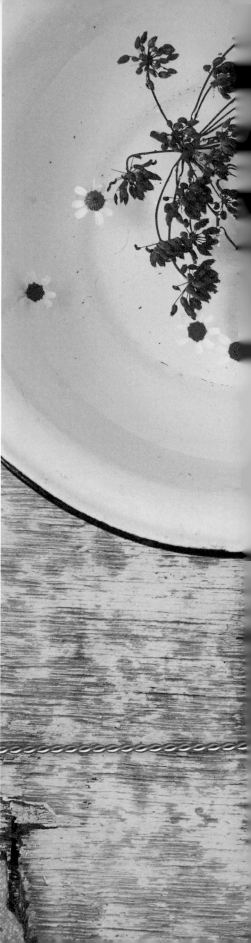

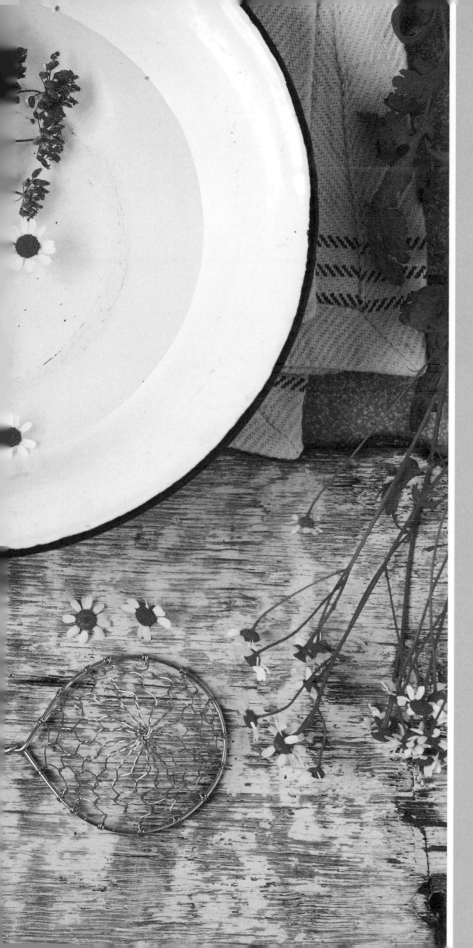

Adaptation:
Decongestant Steam with Ginger and Eucalyptus

In the winter months, the cold winds and harsh weather combined with central heating in our homes can take a toll on our skin. In addition, the inevitable coughs, colds and flu, which seem ever present, can make winter seem like an assault on the senses.

This decongestant steam is based on a traditional treatment that many of us remember from childhood, when we were often given mentholated vapour rubs. The decongestant properties of the ingredients below help to clear the head and chest.

Following the steps for the Facial Steam with Floating Flowers, try adding some of the following essential oils in Step 1 to help relieve blocked sinuses and headaches, as well as assisting with easing cough and cold symptoms: eucalyptus, pine, tea tree, rosemary, lavender, ravensara. You can also add detoxifying and cleansing slices of ginger root, and decongestant juniper if you are lucky enough to have some in your garden.

SAFE STORAGE
Use immediately once you have prepared the steam treatment.

HOW TO APPLY
Inhale the steam through the nose, if possible, to allow the vapour to help relieve congestion in the head.

Dispersing Bath Oil with Dried Flowers and Herbs

This moisturizing, dispersing bath oil can be made simply as a lovely bath soak, or as a decorative item to display in your bathroom with a selection of dried flowers and herbs. A beautiful glass decanter-style bottle is the perfect container for your creative ideas.

Makes approx. 100ml (3½fl oz)

INGREDIENTS
a selection of suitable flowers
   and herbs (see page 18)
25ml (5 tsp) sunflower oil
5ml (1 tsp) evening primrose oil
5ml (1 tsp) rosehip oil
50ml (1½fl oz) sweet almond oil
10ml (2 tsp) Polysorbate 20
60 drops neroli essential oil
20 drops jasmine essential oil in
   dilution
40 drops lemongrass essential oil

SPECIAL EQUIPMENT
sterilized glass bottle and cork
   closure (to suit flowers chosen)
scissors or garden secateurs
tweezers
kitchen towel (paper towel)
tray

SAFE STORAGE
Store in a cool, dry place away from
sunlight. Keeps for up to 6 months
if unopened; or 4 weeks once open.

HOW TO APPLY
Add 2 to 3 tablespoons to your bath.
The moisturizing oils will disperse in the
water, creating a luxurious, scented bath,
which will soften and condition the skin.

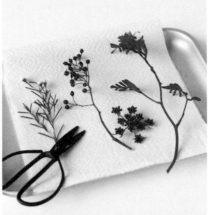

Step 1
Place sheets of kitchen towel (paper towel) on a tray that fits in your airing cupboard, then place your chosen flowers on the tray, ideally with the petals flat. Leave the stalks as long as possible as they can be cut to the desired length later. Leave the tray in the cupboard for up to a week to dry fully. Keep away from strong direct light.

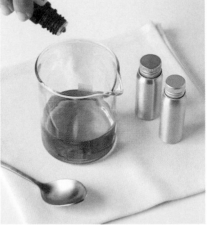

Step 2
Measure the oils and Polysorbate 20 into a glass measuring jug. Add the essential oils and ensure the bath oil is well mixed. Choose a suitable glass bottle in which to display the flowers and herbs inside your oil. The bottle will need to have a wide neck to allow you to place the flowers inside with the aid of long tweezers.

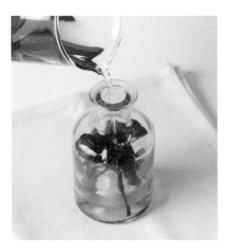

Step 3
Once the flowers are dry (but still pliable), select the most suitable for placing in the bottle. Cut the stems to varying lengths to allow you to position the flower heads at different heights in the bottle for best effect. Using tweezers, gently push the flowers into the bottle – longest first as these anchor any additional flower heads or shorter pieces which may have a tendency to float once the oil is added – then use the tweezers to move them around for the best placing. Pour the prepared bath oil into the bottle so that the flowers are fully covered.

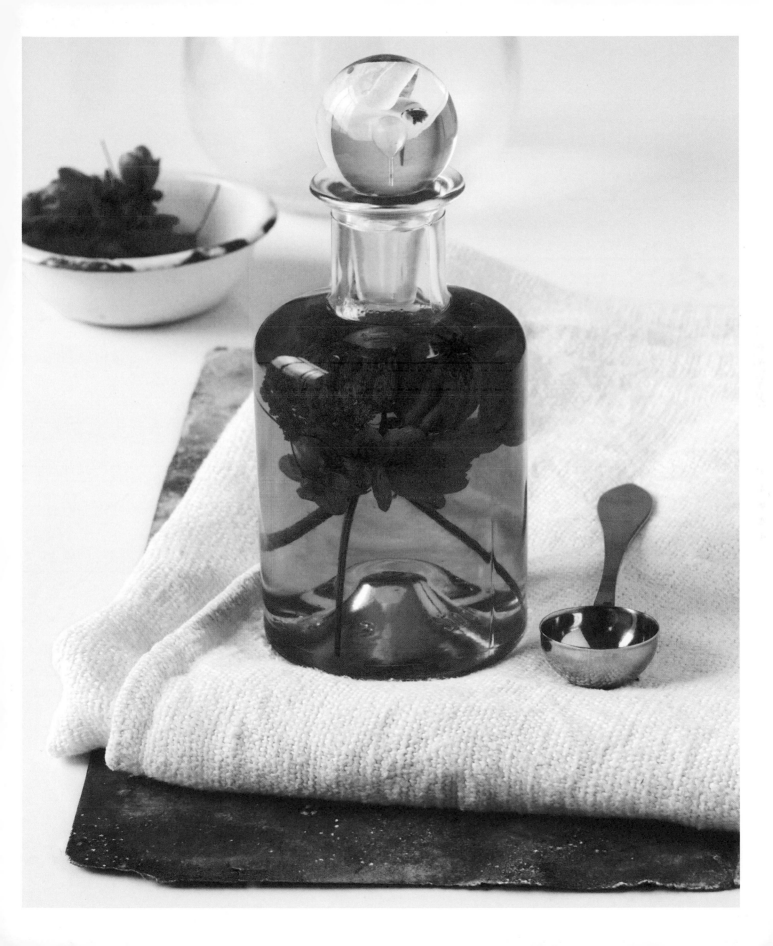

Facial Serum with Pomegranate and Geranium

This regenerating facial serum with pomegranate and geranium is light enough to use underneath make-up, but still packs a punch of rich antioxidant oils to help nourish and protect the skin. Aloe vera juice soothes and calms, while the notes of geranium and frankincense essential oils add just the right fragrant balance to help start your day.

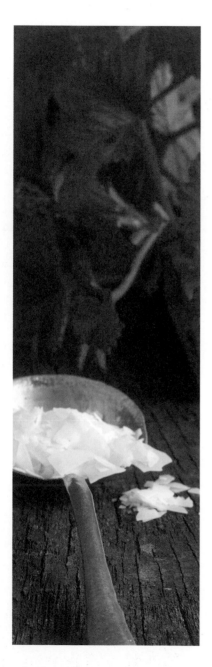

Makes approx. 100ml (3½fl oz)

INGREDIENTS
2ml (½ tsp) glycerine
0.3g (1⁄16 tsp) xanthan gum
80ml (2¾fl oz) aloe vera juice
4ml (¾ tsp) pomegranate oil
4ml (¾ tsp) olive oil
4ml (¾ tsp) Squalane
3g (½ tsp) Olivem 1000
10 drops frankincense essential oil
10 drops geranium essential oil
40 drops grapefruit seed extract

SPECIAL EQUIPMENT
heatproof jug
metal saucepan or bain marie
stick blender
plastic bottle or pump dispenser

SAFE STORAGE
Store in a cool, dry place, away from sunlight. Keeps for up to 3 months.

Step 1
Premix the glycerine with the xanthan gum in a small glass beaker or jug, and stir to ensure there are no lumps. Set aside.

Step 2
Weigh the aloe vera juice, pomegranate oil, olive oil, Squalane and Olivem 1000 into a heatproof jug, and add the premix to the jug. Place the jug in a pan of simmering water or bain marie and heat to 70–80°C (158–176°F); you will need to use a thermometer. Maintain this heat for 30 minutes. To avoid excess evaporation, cover the jug with cling film (plastic wrap).

Step 3
Remove from the heat and whizz with a stick blender. Cool to around 40°C (104°F), add the essential oils and grapefruit seed extract and mix well until uniform. The serum will be quite free-flowing and can be dispensed from either a plastic bottle or a pump dispenser.

HOW TO APPLY
Use at night or in the morning under make-up. Rub a little of the serum between your fingers and apply a light layer to the skin.

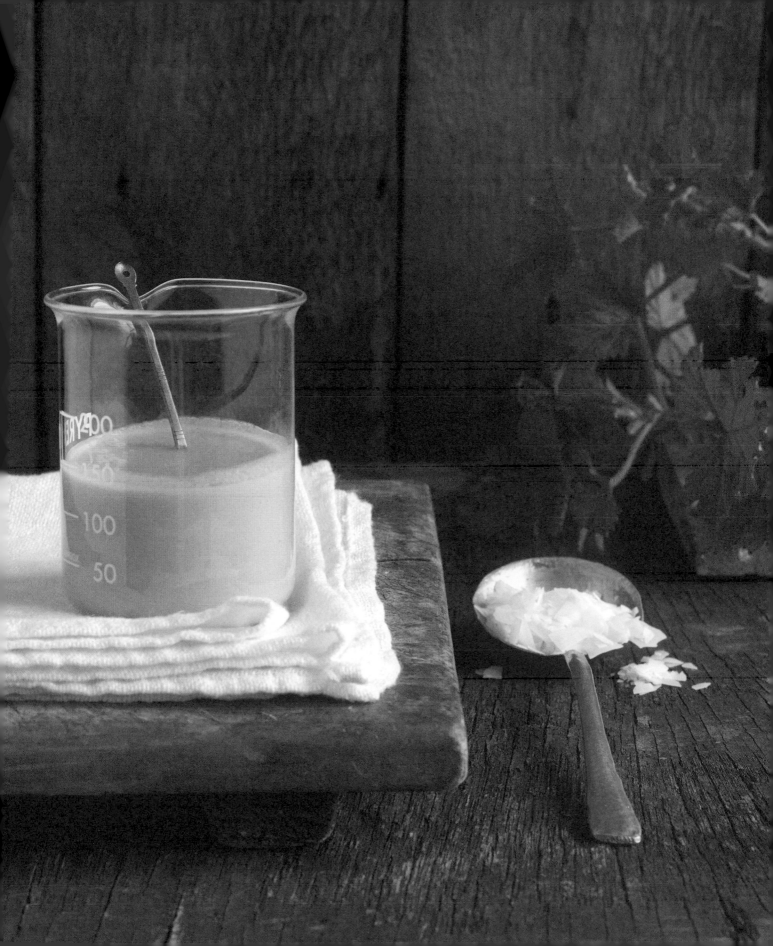

Regenerating Rose Facial Oil

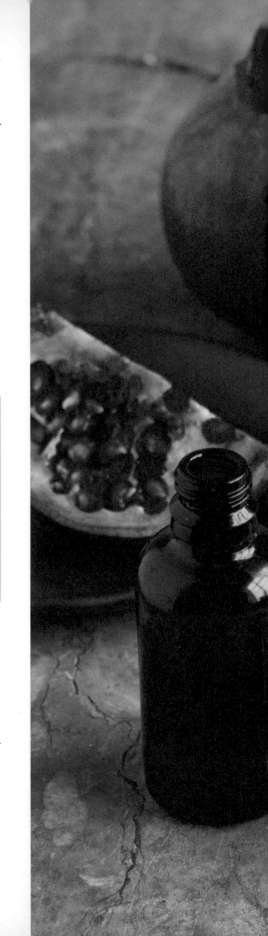

This rich yet light and easily absorbed facial treatment uses a nourishing blend of oils, including rice bran oil. Widely available in supermarkets due to its more common culinary usage, it also has great skincare benefits. Peruvian Inca Inchi, rich in antioxidants and Omega 3, 6 and 9, protects and moisturizes dry skin, while pomegranate oil and rosehip oil offer regenerative and anti-ageing properties. As this recipe contains no water and is simply a mix of beneficial oils, there is no need for heating or a preservative, making it a quick and easy product to make. As well as being a facial oil, you could use this recipe as a facial massage treatment either for someone else, or as a self-massage (see below).

Makes approx. 50ml (1½fl oz)

INGREDIENTS
10ml (2 tsp) Inca Inchi oil
10ml (2 tsp) rosehip oil
20ml (4 tsp) rice bran oil
5ml (1 tsp) vitamin E oil
5ml (1 tsp) pomegranate oil
3 drops rose geranium essential oil

SPECIAL EQUIPMENT
sterilized bottle and cap

SAFE STORAGE
Store in a cool, dry place, away from sunlight. Keeps for up to 6 months.

Step 1
Measure the oils into a glass jug in the order shown in the ingredients above, add the essential oil and stir to combine thoroughly. Pour the liquid into a sterilized bottle and secure the cap. Using a coloured glass bottle such as green, blue or amber will help to protect the oil and prolong its shelf life.

HOW TO APPLY
Use a few drops of the facial oil night or day and massage into the skin until absorbed. Remember to ensure that your hands are warm before pouring a small amount of the oil into your palm. Rub the palms together to spread the oil and then massage into the face and neck using gentle upward movements with the fingertips. Follow the self-massage instructions on page 59 for more detailed instructions.

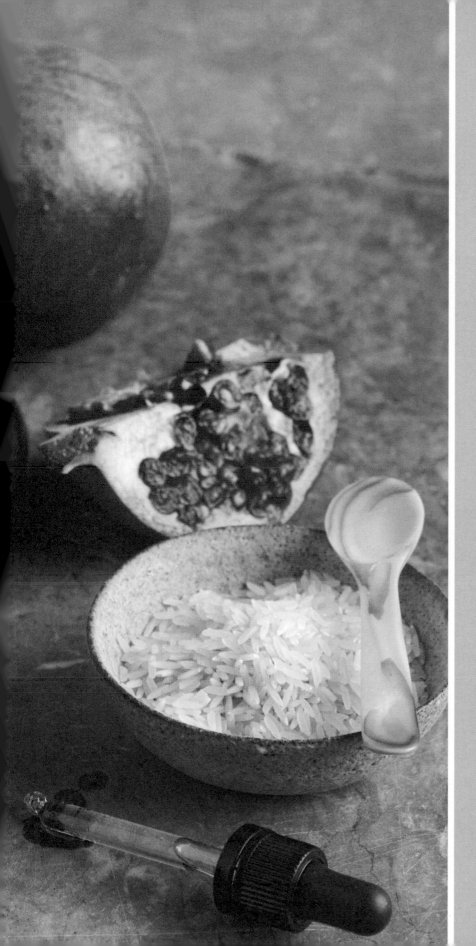

Adaptation:

Restorative Sleep Facial Oil

....

This variation on the Regenerating Rose Facial Oil blends lavender and hop essential oils, known for their ability to assist restful sleep, with regenerative rosehip and moisturizing Inca Inchi and evening primrose oils for a restorative and relaxing bedtime facial treatment.

Makes approx. 50ml (1½fl oz)

INGREDIENTS
10ml (2 tsp) Inca Inchi oil
10ml (2 tsp) rosehip oil
20ml (4 tsp) rice bran oil
5ml (1 tsp) vitamin E oil
5ml (1 tsp) evening primrose oil
3 drops lavender essential oil
2 drops hop essential oil

SPECIAL EQUIPMENT
sterilized bottle and cap

Follow the instructions for the Regenerating Rose Facial Oil.

SAFE STORAGE
Store in a cool, dry place, away from sunlight.
Keeps for up to 6 months.

....

HOW TO APPLY
Use a few drops of the facial oil night or day and massage into the skin until absorbed.

Balancing Body Lotion

This light and easily absorbed body lotion is enriched with nourishing oils and butters to help restore and balance your skin. The scent of orangeflower water combines with exotic ylang and earthy palmarosa essential oils to give that tropical spa sensation. As you apply the lotion, close your eyes and imagine being transported to a lush paradise of palm-fringed beaches, with the sound of gentle waves lapping the shore. It is a real feast for the senses.

Makes approx. 100ml (3½fl oz)

INGREDIENTS

3ml (½ tsp) glycerine
10ml (2 tsp) spring water
60ml (2fl oz) orangeflower water
5g (1 tsp) Olivem 1000
5ml (1 tsp) olive oil
10ml (2 tsp) Inca Inchi oil
6g (1¼ tsp) shea butter
5 drops ylang ylang essential oil
5 drops palmarosa essential oil
40 drops grapefruit seed extract

SPECIAL EQUIPMENT
heatproof jug
metal saucepan or bain marie
thermometer
stick blender
sterilized airtight jar and lid

SAFE STORAGE
Store in a cool, dry place, away from sunlight. Keeps for up to 3 months.

HOW TO APPLY
Apply liberally to the body, especially after a bath or shower. Leave for a few minutes to be absorbed into the skin before getting dressed.

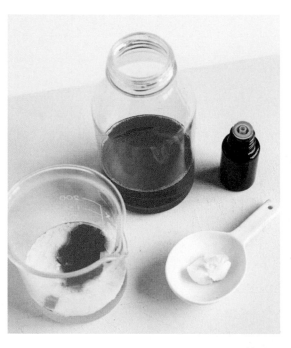

Step 1

Measure all the ingredients except the essential oils and grapefruit seed extract into a heatproof jug. Place the jug in a pan of simmering water or bain marie and heat to 70–80°C (158–176°F); you will need to use a thermometer. Maintain this heat for 30 minutes. To avoid excess evaporation, cover the jug with cling film (plastic wrap). Remove from the heat and whizz with a stick blender.

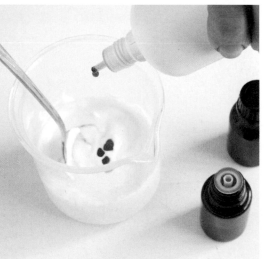

Step 2

Cool to around 40°C (104°F), add the essential oils and grapefruit seed extract and stir until the lotion is uniform. Spoon into a sterilized airtight jar and secure the lid once the mixture has cooled.

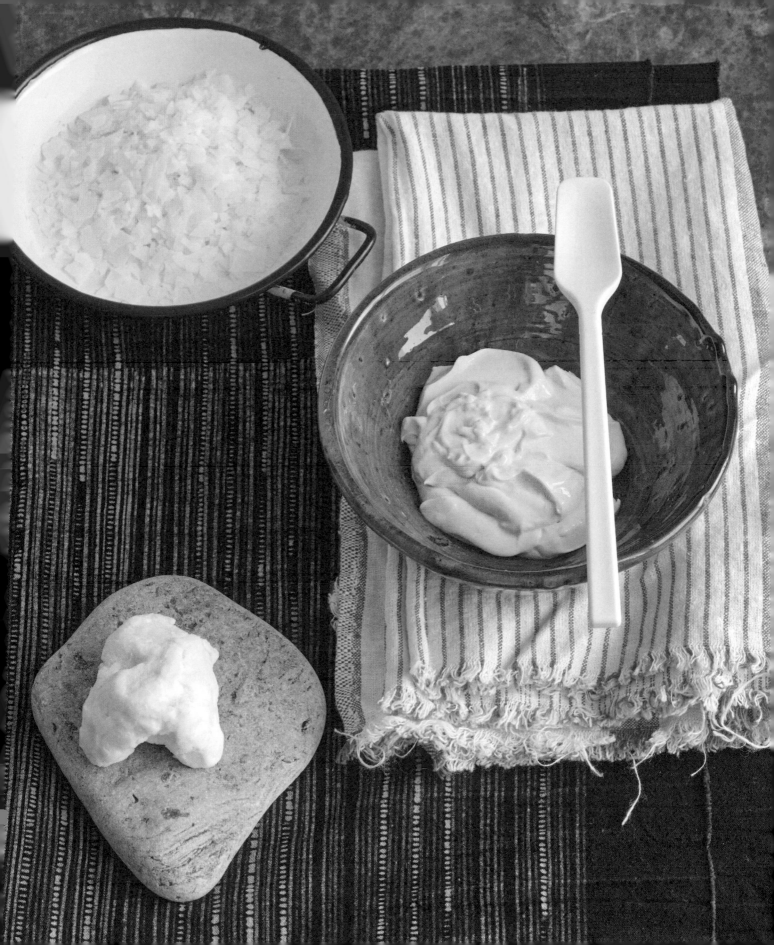

Floating Candles

Floating candles used to be very popular, but in recent years they seem to have become unfashionable, having been ousted by the trend for scented candles in containers. However, floating candles do create the most relaxing and magical ambience when resting on the surface of water in a beautiful bowl. The larger the container, the greater the effect. You can choose a beautifully shaped mould for your candles, add fragrance, a touch of glitter, or embossed patterns to give the candles your own special look. A few well-chosen botanical additions in the water, such as flower heads, or your favourite fresh leaves or herbs, will add to the mood you wish to create.

MATERIALS
natural vegetable-based wax
flowers or foliage, for decoration

SPECIAL EQUIPMENT
bain marie/double boiler (the wax
   could also be melted in a slow
   cooker on low)
thermometer
pouring vessel, such as metal
   teapot with pointed spout
wick, with sustainer, cut to correct
   length and size for your chosen
   mould
wick stickers
mini metal patisserie moulds
large ceramic or glass bowl
optional: wooden skewers
optional: embossing stamps and
   glitter or embossing powder

Tips
*See the tips on page 68 for the Scented
Candles. Please bear these in mind when
working with the candle wax for the
Floating Candles.*

PREPARATION

- Cover work area with an old cloth or newspaper to catch any drips or spillages of wax.
- Wear an apron to protect your clothing from wax spillages.
- Make sure your moulds are clean and dry.
- Measure the volume of your chosen container with water and weigh out the same amount of wax.
- Cut up the wax into smaller pieces if necessary; this will help the wax to melt evenly.
- Choose any embossing stamps or glitter you wish to try.

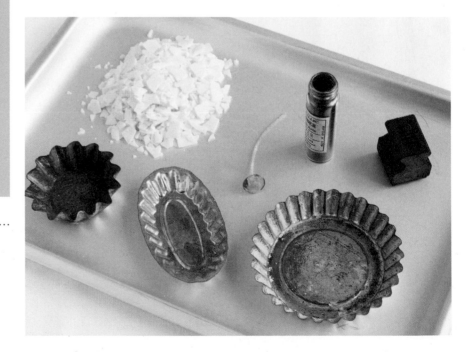

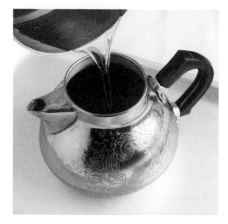

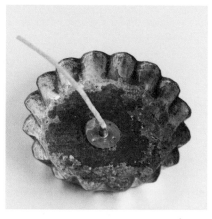

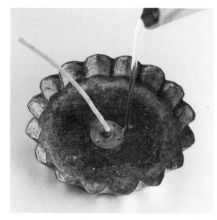

Step 1

Place the wax into the top pan of a bain marie/double boiler. Keep an eye on the water level and do not allow it to boil dry. Once melted, check the temperature of the wax: it should be 60°C (140°F) or just below, but check the instructions supplied with the wax for the recommended pouring temperature. Remove from the heat and leave to cool if necessary. Warm the jug or pourer with hot water, and dry the inside before pouring the wax into the warm pourer.

Step 2

Place a wick sticker centrally in the base of each mould, then place the wick sustainer on top and secure in place. Check the wick is straight. If necessary, place wooden skewers crosswise around the wick to keep it straight.

Step 3

Carefully pour the wax from the pourer into the moulds, all the way to the top if they are relatively shallow. Keep the remaining wax warm over a low heat to top up if the floating candles show signs of dipping in the centre.

Leave to set fully before turning out the candles from the moulds. Fill your bowl two-thirds full with water and arrange the candles with flowers or foliage in the bowl.

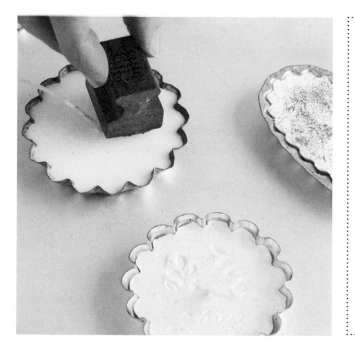

EMBOSSING AND DECORATING (OPTIONAL)

You can choose to decorate your floating candles by creating a relief pattern using embossing stamps if you wish. This will need to be done when the candle wax is almost solid, and it is a case of trial and error to get the wax to the stage where it is still just soft enough to take the emboss (but not too soft!). Use your chosen stamps to gently press an imprint into the candle in the mould. The effect can be enhanced by using embossing powder or extremely fine glitter very sparingly. Again, test out different ideas and products to achieve your desired effect; it does look stunning once the candles are lit and floating in their beautiful bowl.

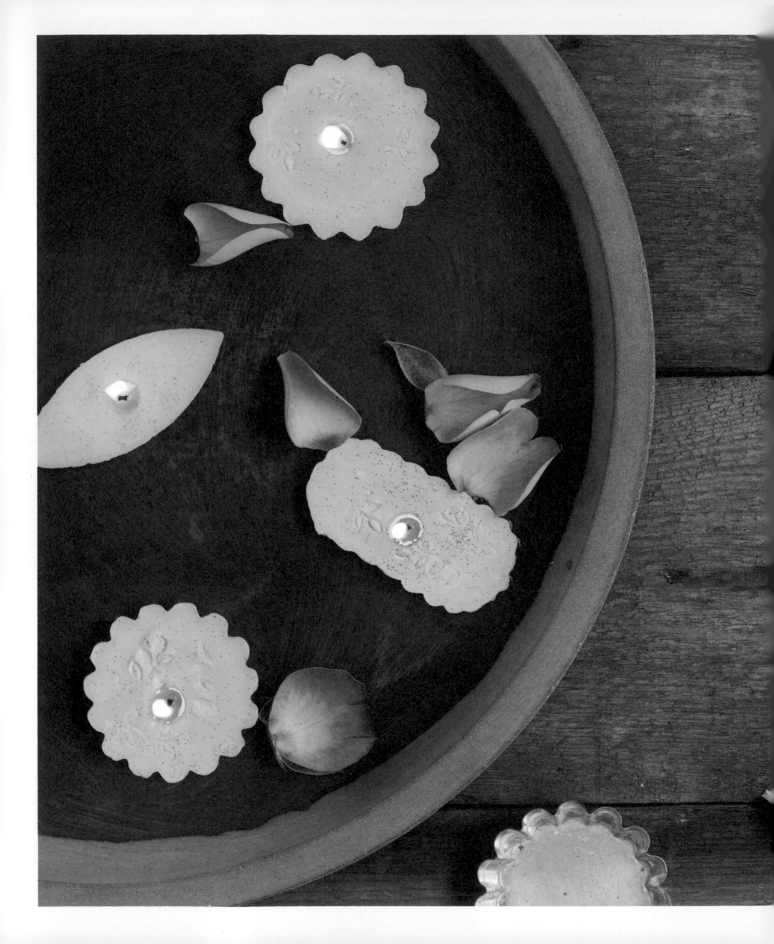

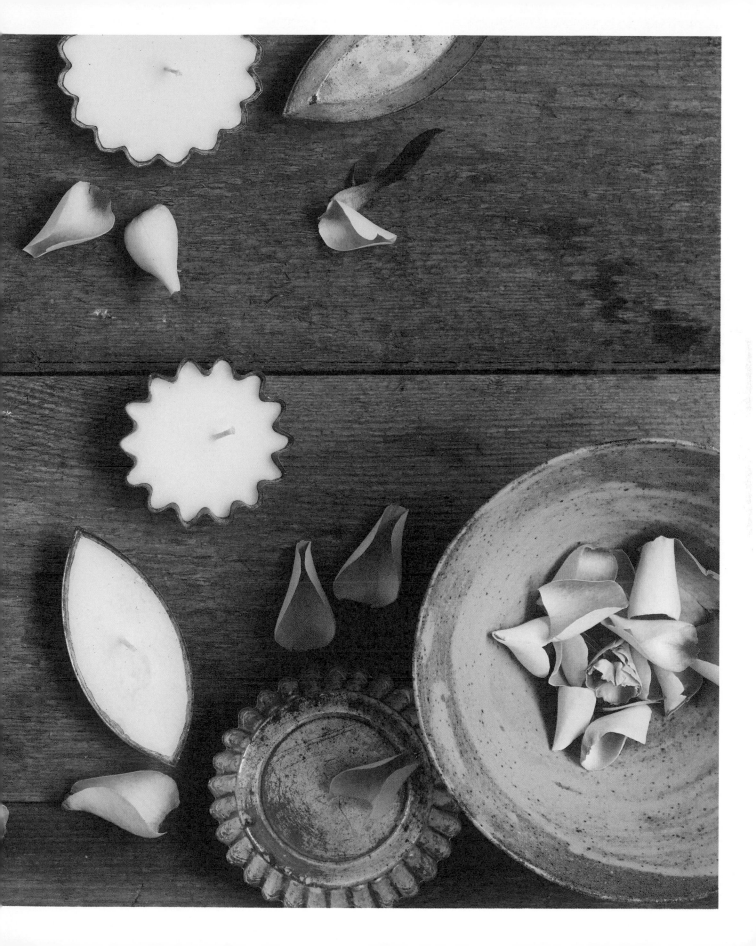

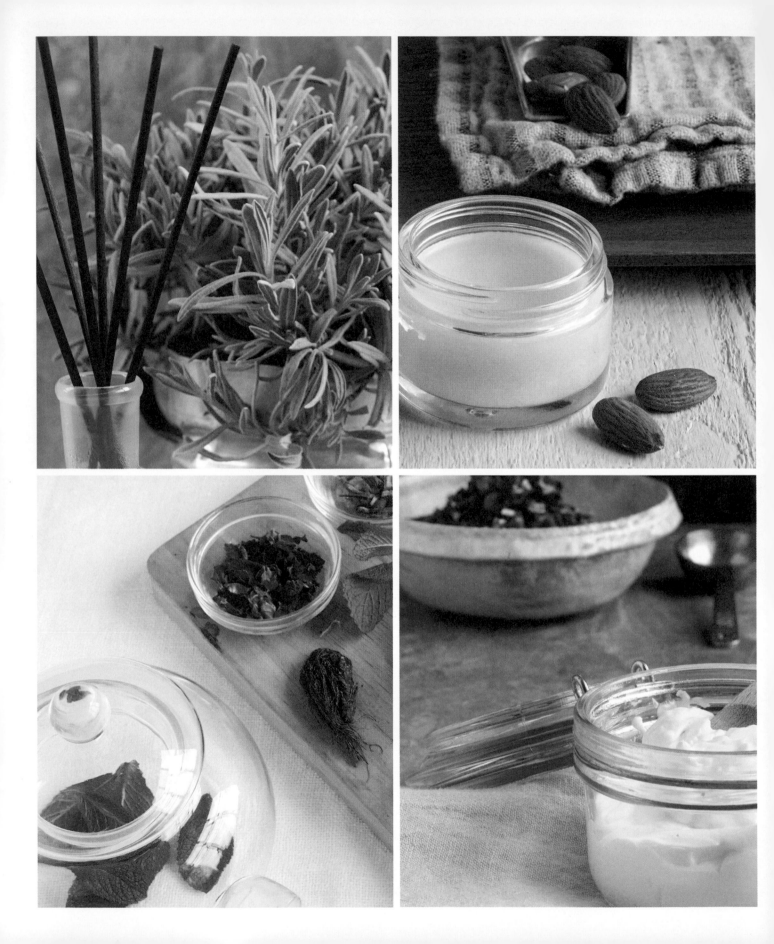

Calming, Sleep-inducing, Restful

HERBAL ESSENTIAL OILS SUCH AS LAVENDER AND HOP HAVE BEEN USED FOR GENERATIONS TO HELP RELAX AND PROMOTE SLEEP. THESE TRIED AND TESTED INGREDIENTS ARE COMBINED WITH CALMING WOODY OILS SUCH AS CEDAR AND SANDALWOOD TO CREATE RELAXING TREATMENTS FOR BOTH BODY AND MIND.

Calming Facial Cleansing Balm

A good cleanser is the key to any spa facial treatment. This solid cleansing balm is the most moisturizing and indulgent facial cleanser, as it melts on the skin, turning to a soft milky lotion as you add warm water. For an exfoliating treatment, add a small amount of bamboo powder to the cleansing balm and combine with your fingers; this is perfect for use on dry skin patches around the elbows, feet and knees. You will find that a little of the cleansing balm goes a long way when using this recipe, making it a great choice for packing in your holiday luggage. At the final stage, why not try pouring some of the product into a separate small plastic jar, specifically for use when travelling. Then you will always be ready with the perfect-sized cleanser if you are packing in a hurry or have limited space in your luggage. The Directory of Suppliers (see page 142) will help you find something suitable.

Makes approx. 100ml (3½fl oz)

INGREDIENTS
40ml (2¾ tbsp) sweet almond oil
10g (2 tsp) Polysorbate 20
38ml (2½ tbsp) fractionated
 coconut oil
5g (1 tsp) cetyl alcohol
6g (1¼ tsp) beeswax
20 drops lavender essential oil

SPECIAL EQUIPMENT
heatproof jug
metal saucepan or bain marie
thermometer
sterilized jars and lids

SAFE STORAGE
Store in a cool, dry place, away from sunlight. Keeps for up to 6 months.

HOW TO APPLY
Scoop out about half a teaspoonful and, using the fingertips, massage the balm gently around the face to loosen make-up. Remove the residue with a Hot Cloth Facial Cleanser (see page 54) for super clean and calmed skin.

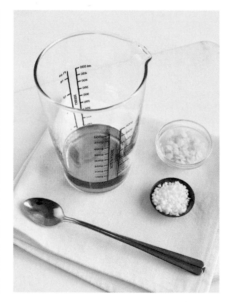

Step 1
Place all the ingredients apart from the lavender essential oil in a heatproof jug and place the jug in a pan of simmering water or bain marie. Heat to 70–80°C (158–176°F); you will need to use a thermometer. Remove the jug from the heat and leave to cool slightly, then whizz with a stick blender.

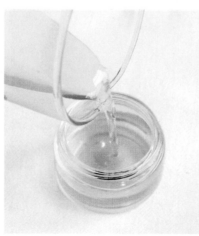

Step 2
Allow the temperature of the liquid to reduce to 45–50°C (113–122°F), then stir in the lavender oil to combine. Pour the liquid balm into sterilized jars and allow to set, then seal the lids.

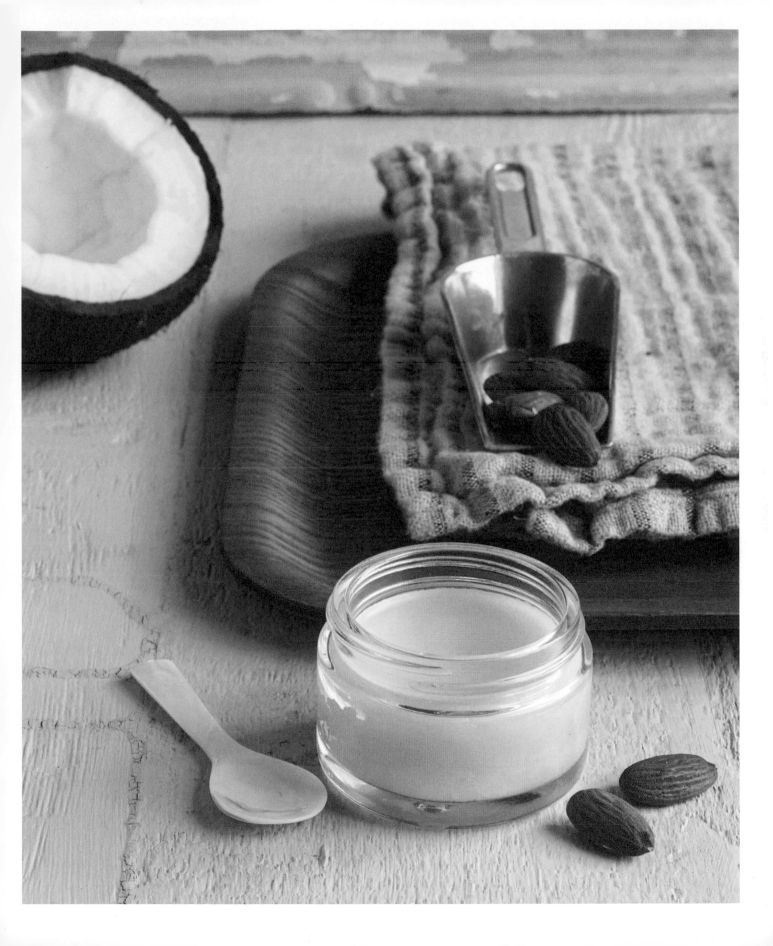

Rich, Restful Night Cream Mask

A rich and nourishing night-time treat to soothe and smooth fatigued skin. Allow the beneficial butters, plant oils and essential oils to get to work while you sleep.

Makes approx. 100ml (3½fl oz)

INGREDIENTS

Phase 1

43ml (3 tbsp) lavender water

5ml (1 tsp) aloe juice

10g (2 tsp) ESP Organic SafeEmuls SCA

5g (1 tsp) shea butter

5g (1 tsp) cetearyl alcohol

2g (½ tsp) beeswax

Phase 2

7ml (1½ tsp) rosehip oil

7ml (1½ tsp) evening primrose oil

14ml (3 tsp) wheatgerm oil

Phase 3

15 drops lavender essential oil

5 drops hop essential oil

40 drops grapefruit seed extract

SPECIAL EQUIPMENT

heatproof jug

metal saucepan or bain marie

thermometer

stick blender

SAFE STORAGE

Store in a cool, dry place, away from sunlight. Keeps for up to 3 months.

Step 1

Place all the ingredients from phase 1 into a heatproof jug. Place the jug in a pan of simmering water or bain marie and heat to 70–80°C (158–176°F); you will need to use a thermometer. Maintain this heat for 30 minutes. To avoid excess evaporation, cover the jug with cling film (plastic wrap).

Step 2

Remove the jug from the heat and allow to cool slightly. Add the phase 2 ingredients and whizz with a stick blender until a cream is formed. Allow the temperature to reduce to 40°C (104°F), then stir in the phase 3 ingredients and continue mixing until the cream is smooth and uniform.

HOW TO APPLY

Apply generously to the face and neck and massage into the skin (see page 59 for self-massage techniques). Leave overnight and remove with cleanser in the morning.

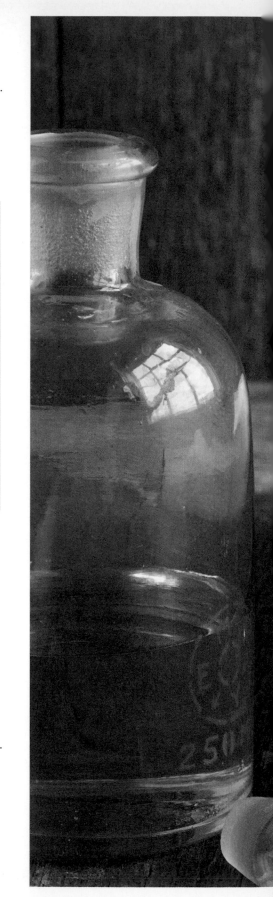

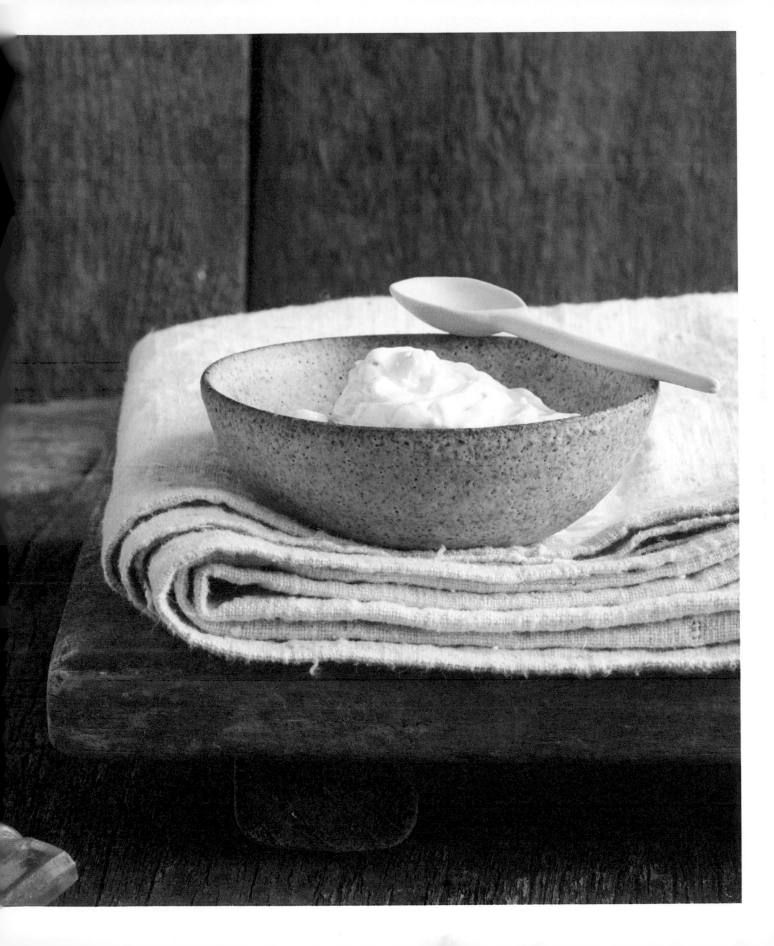

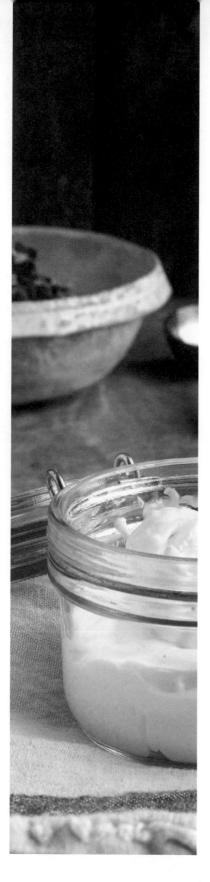

Relaxing Herbal Body Cream

A luxurious and indulgent body cream enriched with nourishing rosehip and argan oils blended with shea butter to pamper, soothe and help calm tired and troubled skin. A blend of lavender, sandalwood and geranium essential oils provides just the right relaxing and mood-enhancing scent.

Makes approx. 100ml (3½fl oz)

INGREDIENTS
12g (2½ tsp) ESP Organic SafeEmuls SCA
5ml (1 tsp) glycerine
60ml (2fl oz) lavender water
5ml (1 tsp) rosehip oil
5ml (1 tsp) argan oil
9g (1¾ tsp) shea butter
2g (½ tsp) cetyl alcohol
8 drops lavender essential oil
4 drops sandalwood essential oil
8 drops geranium essential oil
40 drops grapefruit seed extract

SPECIAL EQUIPMENT
heatproof jug
metal saucepan or bain marie
thermometer
stick blender
sterilized airtight jars with lids

SAFE STORAGE
Store in a cool, dry place, away from sunlight. Keeps for up to 3 months.

Step 1
Place all the ingredients apart from the essential oils and grapefruit seed extract in a heatproof jug. Place the jug in a pan of simmering water and heat to 70–80°C (158–176°F); you will need to use a thermometer. Maintain this heat for 30 minutes. To avoid excess evaporation, cover the jug with cling film (plastic wrap).

Step 2
Remove the jug from the heat and allow to cool slightly, then whizz with a stick blender. Allow the temperature to reduce to 40°C (104°F), then add the essential oils and grapefruit seed extract. Spoon into sterilized airtight jars and secure the lids once the mixture has completely cooled.

HOW TO APPLY
Apply liberally to the body, especially after a bath or shower. Leave for a few minutes to be absorbed into the skin before getting dressed.

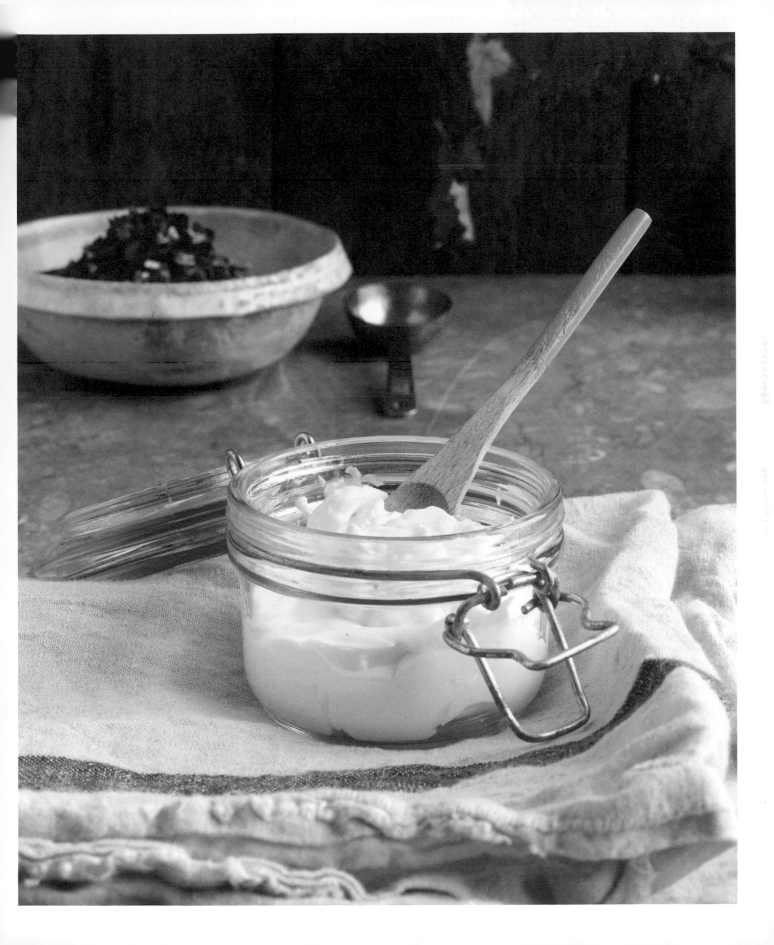

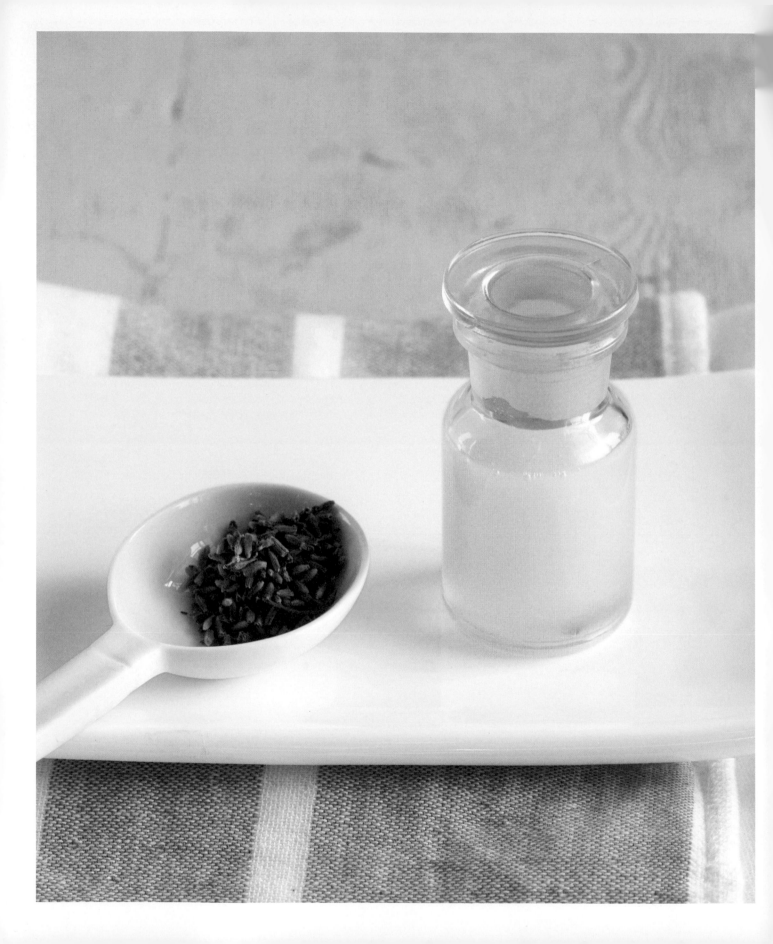

Indulgent Moisturizing Bath Soak with Lavender

This highly concentrated and super moisturizing bath soak contains only natural foaming agents to give the bath water a soft, foamy texture, as well as soothing evening primrose oil and relaxing lavender oil to give your skin a truly pampering and hydrating bathtime treat. This kind of richly indulgent recipe is one you would struggle to find in a commercial product due to the expensive ingredients used, so it really makes sense to have a go at making this yourself. Once you have tried it you will really understand the difference and return to the recipe time after time.

Makes approx. 100ml (3½fl oz)

INGREDIENTS
10ml (2 tsp) evening primrose oil
56ml (1¾fl oz) Sucragel CF
28ml (1¾ tbsp) coco-glucoside
6ml (1¼ tsp) lavender essential
  oil

SPECIAL EQUIPMENT
sterilized bottle and cap

SAFE STORAGE
Store in a cool, dry place, away from sunlight. Keeps for up to 3 months.

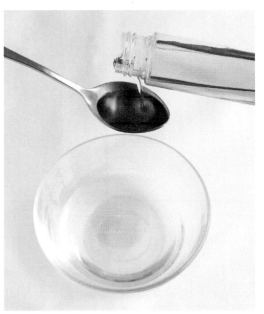

Step 1
In a small glass dish or beaker, measure out the evening primrose oil into the Sucragel CF and stir carefully to combine this premix.

Step 2
Slowly stir through the coco-glucoside and lavender essential oil in turn until the mix is completely uniform. Pour into a sterilized bottle and seal.

HOW TO APPLY
Use sparingly, as this recipe is really concentrated: pour a couple of teaspoons into a bath of warm running water to disperse.

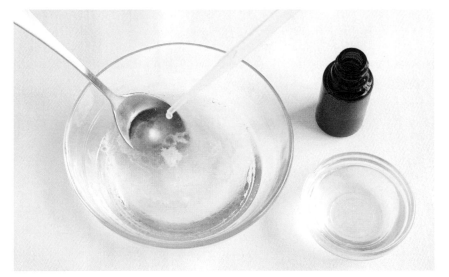

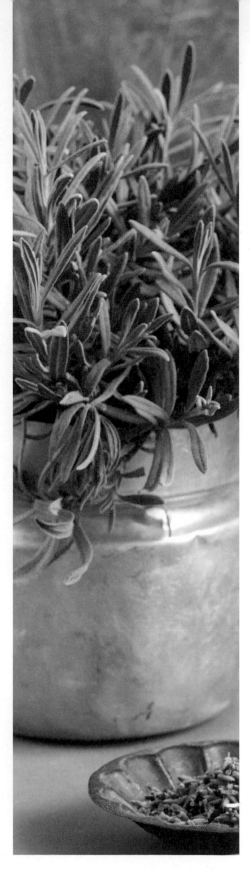

Relaxing and Calming Reed Diffuser

Many of us have trouble sleeping, but there are a few simple ideas which can help us to relax and switch off. Essential oils are powerful tools that can aid in dealing with the pressures of daily life, and this reed diffuser, with its relaxing and restful essential oil blend, is a really useful item to make for your home spa.

Makes approx. 50ml (1½fl oz)

INGREDIENTS
34ml (2¼ tbsp) formulator's alcohol
75 drops lavender essential oil
30 drops cedarwood essential oil
30 drops amyris essential oil
15 drops cypress essential oil
8.5ml (1½ tsp) deionized water

SPECIAL EQUIPMENT
rattan reed sticks
narrow-necked bottle with seal

SAFE STORAGE
This recipe is sufficient for a 50ml (1½fl oz) diffuser, which should last for around 6 weeks, but you can double the quantities and make 100ml (3½fl oz), which will last for around 3 months. We generally prefer to make a smaller amount as the mixture stays fresh and is less likely to be contaminated by dust or any airborne particles that could settle in the bottle.

Step 1
Measure the formulators' alcohol into a beaker, then add the essential oils and stir until clear. Slowly add the deionized water, and mix thoroughly. Pour the liquid into a suitable bottle, seal, and allow to macerate in a cool place for a few days prior to using the diffuser.

Step 2
When ready, remove the seal and insert around 4 to 6 rattan reeds into the bottle.

HOW TO USE
Turn the reeds regularly to ensure that the fragrant liquid travels up the length of the reeds and disperses into the air.

Safety Tips
The bottle should not be too tall, as it could be knocked over. Diffusers which contain alcohol and essential oils are flammable and can be damaging to furnishings and painted surfaces. Ensure that diffusers are placed well away from children, pets and open flames.

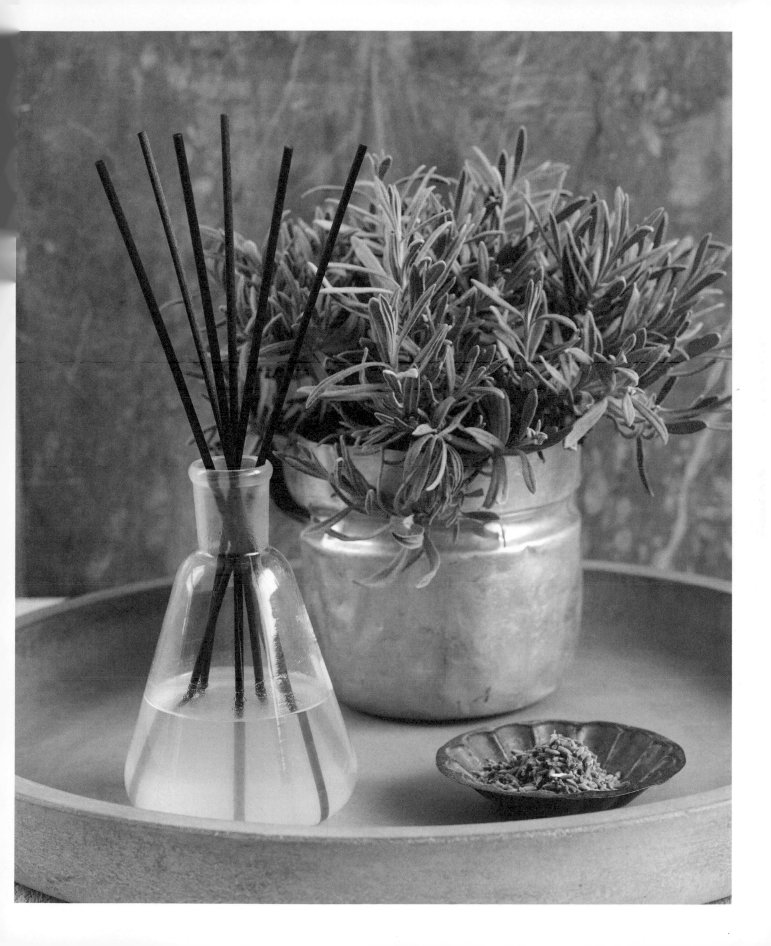

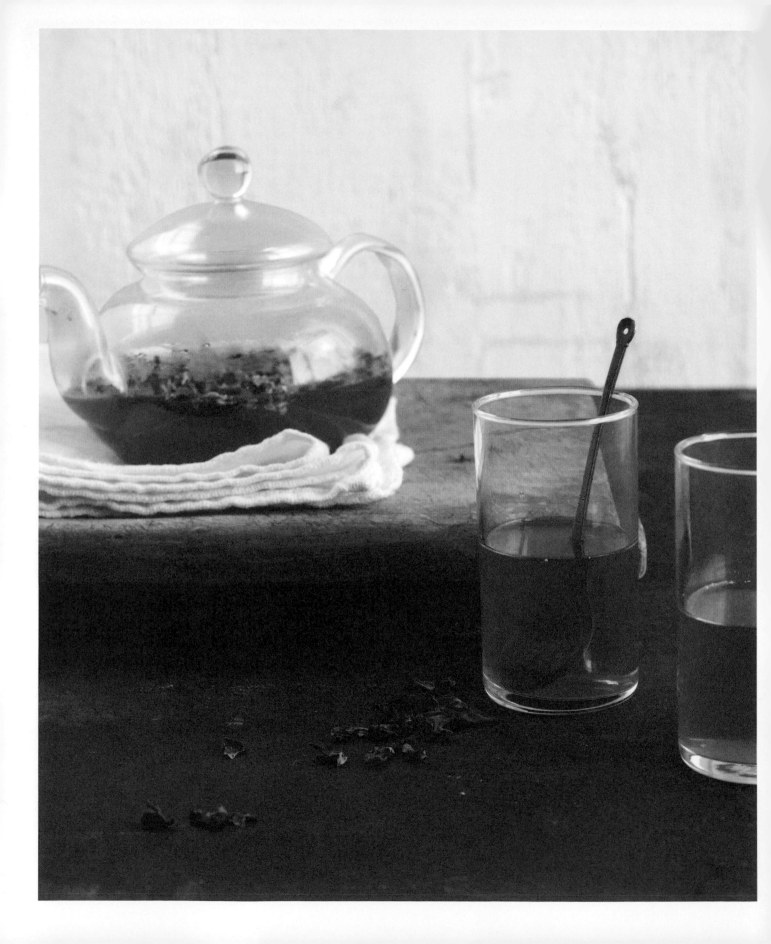

Sleepy Herbal Tea Infusion

Caffeine is the last thing you need if you want to get a good night's sleep, so any evening drink should avoid traditional tea and coffee which might stimulate the system. This recipe contains valerian and lime flowers, which are known for their ability to relax and aid restful sleep, and liquorice and mint, both of which are helpful for digestion. You will find that using whole, dried ingredients as well as fresh herbs creates a much finer tasting tea than anything you might find in a sachet, where the ingredients are finely cut and chopped.

Makes approx. 2 cups

FRESH INGREDIENTS
3 sprigs of peppermint or spearmint, or more or less as desired

DRY INGREDIENTS
1 piece of valerian root, approx. 2.5–3.75cm (1–1½in) long, crushed
5g (1 tsp) liquorice root, chopped
5g (1 tsp) lime flowers
5g (1 tsp) rose petals

SPECIAL EQUIPMENT
glass teapot
kettle
tea strainer
2 cups, mugs or tea glasses

SAFE STORAGE
The tea should be enjoyed immediately and should not be stored for future use.

HOW TO USE
The tea is best enjoyed hot, so serve immediately.

Tip!
If you make the tea in a glass teapot you will be able to see just how beautiful the colours of the ingredients look, which is also part of the holistic experience.

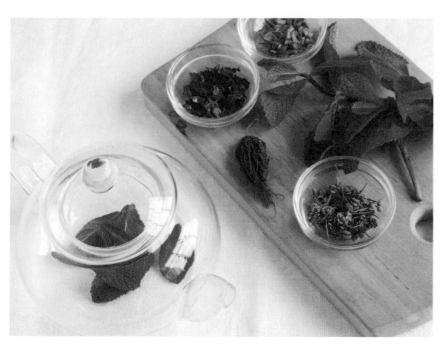

Step 1
Pick your fresh ingredients and wash them, then set aside.

Step 2
Measure out the dry ingredients into a teapot and add the mint. Pour over boiling water sufficient for two cups. Allow to infuse for 5 to 10 minutes before pouring into the cups through a strainer. No sweetener is required as the liquorice gives a natural sweet aspect to the tea.

Lavender and Hop Pillow Mist

Both lavender and hops have traditionally been used to soothe and calm, and in particular to help promote rest and relaxed slumber. Hop pillows, made using English hops, are well known for their association with helping you to drift off and get a good night's sleep. This atomizer mist is a simple but effective way to add calming aromas for a more restful sleep experience. You will need to choose a bottle with a very fine atomizer pump, like those used for perfume, so that the mist lightly scents the pillow, rather than making it too wet.

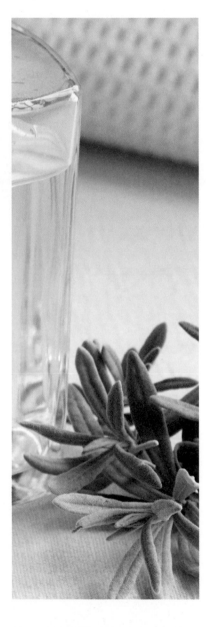

Makes approx. 100ml (3½fl oz)

INGREDIENTS
76ml (2½fl oz) formulators' alcohol
2 drops lavender essential oil
3 drops hop essential oil
24ml (1½ tbsp) spring water or
  demineralized water

SPECIAL EQUIPMENT
glass storage bottle with cap
optional: coffee filter paper
glass or plastic bottle with atomizer
  spray

SAFE STORAGE
Store in a cool, dry place, away from sunlight. Keeps for up to 3 months.

Step 1
Pour the formulators' alcohol into a glass jug or beaker, then add the lavender and hop essential oils, stirring until clear. Finally, add the spring or demineralized water slowly, and stir to mix thoroughly.

Step 2
Transfer the liquid into the glass storage bottle, seal the cap and leave in a cool place to mature for 5 to 7 days to allow the essential oils to settle.

Step 3
After maturing, chill the liquid overnight in the fridge, then decant into a spray bottle. If desired, decant the liquid through a fine coffee filter paper to remove any particles. Finally, attach the cap.

HOW TO APPLY
Spray a small amount on to your pillow at bedtime and allow the aroma of lavender and hops to help you sleep.

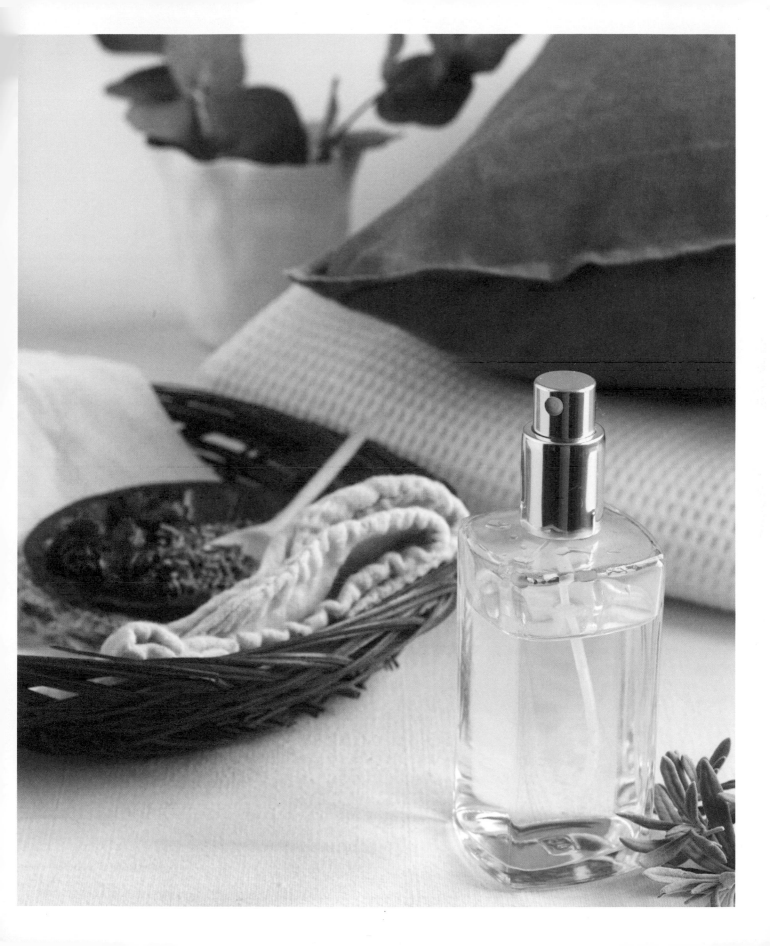

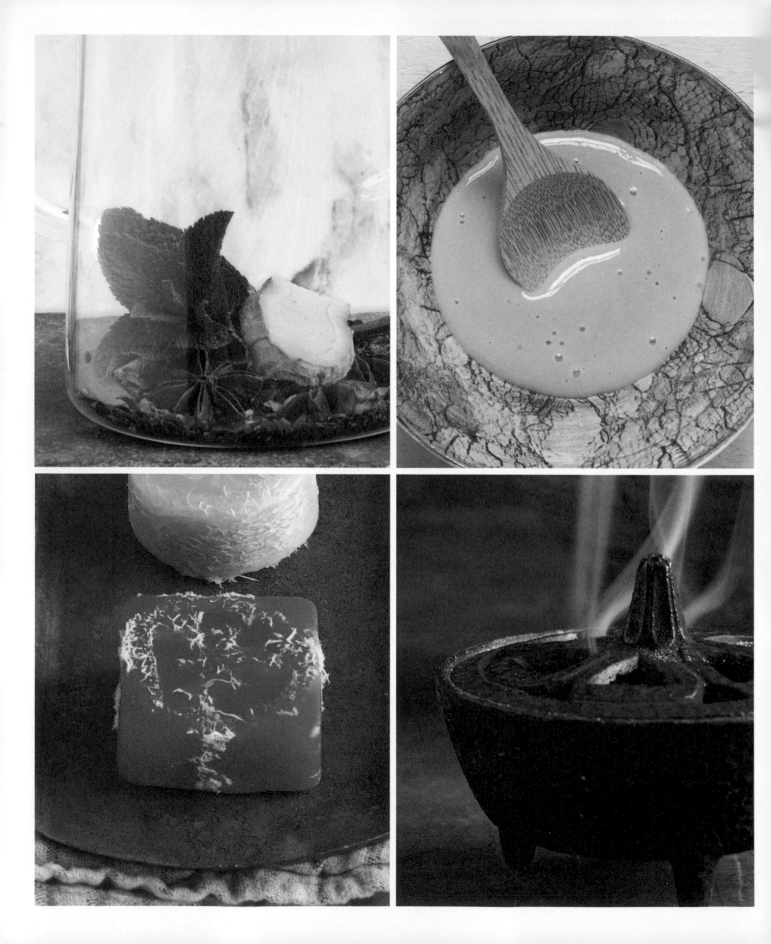

Detoxifying, Cleansing

FRESH, CITRUSY LIME, LEMONGRASS AND MELISSA
JOIN AROMATIC PLANT OILS OF CYPRESS
AND FENNEL, AS WELL AS OZONIC SEAWEED,
TO CREATE A SELECTION OF DETOXIFYING
TREATMENTS DESIGNED TO CLEANSE AND KICK-
START THE BODY AND ELIMINATE TOXINS.

Peeling Seaweed Face Mask

This peelable face mask is both fun to use and highly effective. It uses a seaweed alginate base, which is packed with minerals that activate the mask to set on contact with water, giving your face a cool, revitalizing experience. To this we have added camomile tea to give a soothing, calming quality to the detoxifying effect of the seaweed.

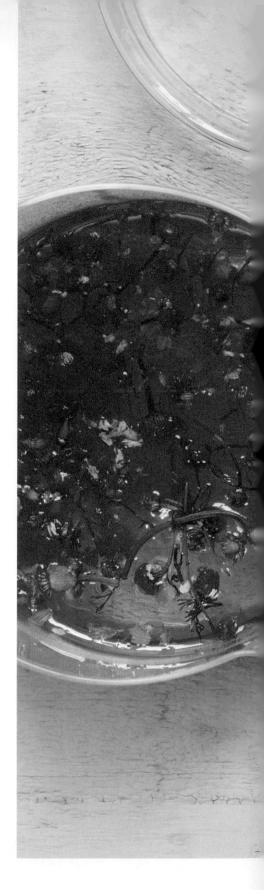

Makes approx. 50g (1½oz)

INGREDIENTS
40ml (2¾ tbsp) camomile tea, made
  using camomile flower tea bags
  (such as teapigs)
10g (2 tsp) alginate powder

SPECIAL EQUIPMENT
heatproof jug
tall ceramic mug
broad-bladed knife or palette knife

SAFE STORAGE
The mask should be used immediately and any excess discarded after use. Do not discard down the sink as the alginate does not dissolve in water; discard with household waste or as composting.

Step 1
Make up the camomile tea in the heatproof jug following the instructions on the packet. Leave to cool completely.

Step 2
Place the alginate powder in the ceramic mug and add the cold tea, mixing quickly and continuously with the palette knife to form a smooth, runny paste. Mash the mix against the sides of the mug to break up any undispersed powder. As soon as the tea is added to the alginate powder the setting process begins, so speed of mixing and application to the face (see below) is crucial for effective results.

HOW TO APPLY
Apply a thick layer of the mask to the face immediately and allow to set; this will take only a few minutes. Leave for 10–15 minutes, then peel the mask off; it should come off in large pieces or as one continuous film. Discard in household waste.

Variation
For a cooling eye mask, pour the mix into two dessertspoons and allow to set. Remove the set gel from the spoons and place over or around closed eyes. Relax and enjoy.

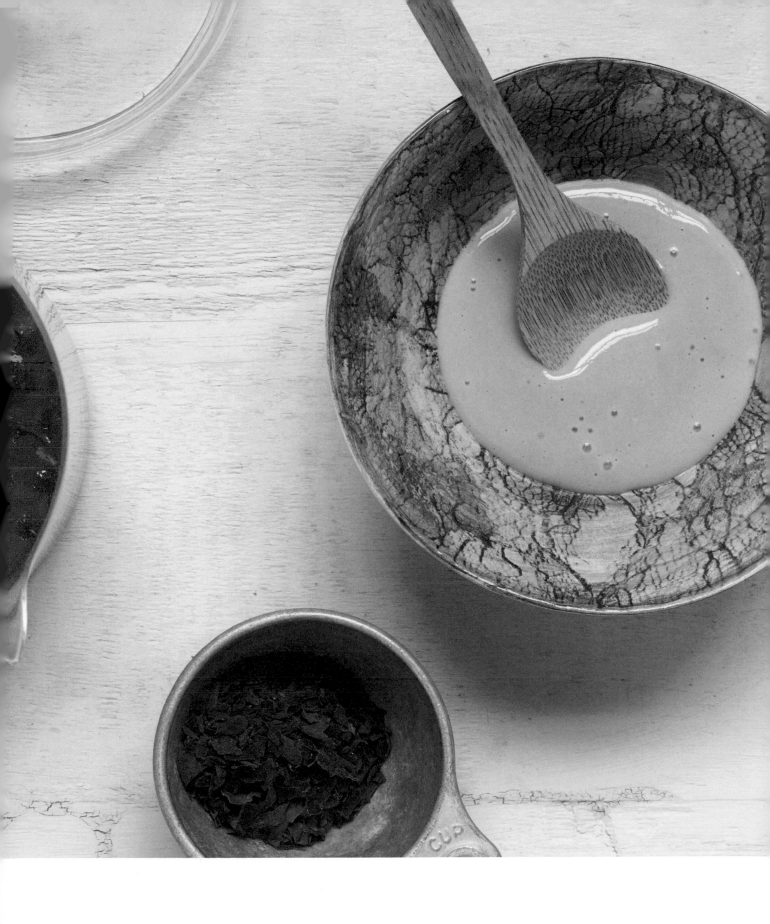

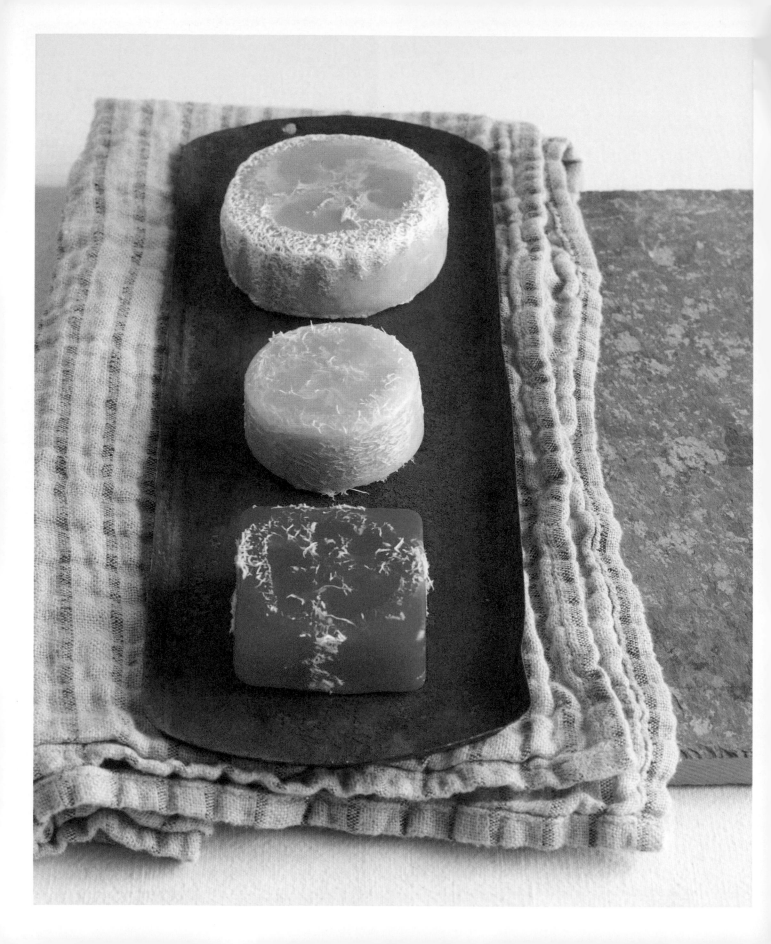

Ginger, Lemongrass and Lime Loofah Soap

The fresh, zesty fragrance from the ginger, lemongrass and lime essential oils makes a really refreshing addition to this exfoliating treatment. This is a very simple and quick way to make your own soap, and this particular form of melt-and-pour base is a clear, vegetable-derived version. Adding a loofah into your soap mould with the melt-and-pour base transforms this from simply a soap to an exfoliating treatment ideal for use in the bath or shower. You can also have fun adding your own colour, if you wish. If you do choose to colour your soap, take care to add the concentrated colour very gradually, to avoid ending up with a more vibrant shade than you had intended.

Makes 1 loofah soap

INGREDIENTS
100g (3½oz) Crystal Clear Melt
    and Pour Soap Base
optional: natural food colouring
6 drops ginger essential oil
7 drops lemongrass essential oil
7 drops lime essential oil

SPECIAL EQUIPMENT
silicone mould or shallow dish
loofah slice, size and shape to suit
    your mould (see Step 1)
cling film (plastic wrap)
heatproof jug
metal saucepan or bain marie

SAFE STORAGE
*Store in a cool, dry place, away from
sunlight. Keeps for up to 6 months.*

HOW TO APPLY
*Use the loofah soap as you would a
conventional soap, working a lather into
the hands and paying attention to areas
of hard skin, allowing the loofah to gently
exfoliate as you wash.*

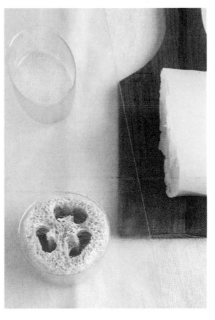

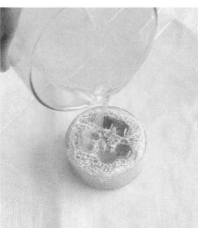

Step 1

Choose a suitable mould or dish, approximately the same diameter as the loofah, and place the loofah inside. A silicone mould is the best option, but if you cannot find one then choose a shallow dish and line it with a large sheet of cling film (plastic wrap), which overlaps the sides of the container. Keep the cling film (plastic wrap) smooth with no creases. Cut the soap base into small pieces, approx. 2.5 × 2.5cm (1 × 1in). Place in a heatproof jug in a bain marie over a low heat and warm the soap base until melted, then remove from the heat and add the food colouring (if using), a couple of drops at a time, until you reach the desired shade.

Step 2

Cool the soap to around 60°C (140°F); you will notice a skin beginning to form on the top. Add the essential oils and stir to combine. Pour the soap into the prepared mould and allow to cool and solidify completely. Release the soap from the mould carefully by turning it over and pulling gently on the cling film (plastic wrap) to ease it out.

Detoxifying Fizzing Seaweed Bath Tablets

Makes approx. 225g (8oz)

INGREDIENTS

10g (2 tsp) dried fresh seaweed
125g (4oz) sodium bicarbonate
62g (2¼ oz) citric acid
25g (1oz) cornflour
2.5ml (½ tsp) essential oil blend
  (see below)
witch hazel, as required (see
  method)

Essential Oil Blend
20 drops grapefruit essential oil
18 drops cedarwood essential oil
12 drops palmarosa essential oil

SPECIAL EQUIPMENT
colander
metal baking tray
coffee grinder/smoothie blender
plastic pipette
spray bottle/atomizer
vinyl gloves
vintage patisserie moulds
optional: garlic press

SAFE STORAGE
*Store the tablets in an airtight jar
for up to 6 weeks.*

HOW TO APPLY
*Place 2 or 3 tablets in a warm bath
and allow the fizzy tablets to soften and
fragrance the bath water. The essential oils
will mix with the aroma of seaweed for a
fabulous, detoxifying soak.*

These fun, refreshing alternatives to bath bombs are quick and simple to create and can be varied in shape and size depending on your choice of mould. To use a garlic press to make the tablets, cut a piece of greaseproof paper to fit the base of the press, add the powder into the press and place a second identical piece of paper on top. Press down to make a tablet and leave for a few minutes before turning out. We have used freshly harvested seaweed for its detoxifying properties, but seaweed powder is also suitable.

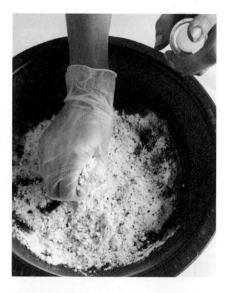

Step 1
Preheat the oven to 120°C (250°F). Place the seaweed in a colander and rinse with plenty of clean, running water. Place the seaweed on a baking tray and into the oven for about 30 minutes until completely dry. Remove from the oven and set aside to cool, then blitz the seaweed in a coffee grinder until the particles are fine. Weigh the other dry ingredients into a mixing bowl, along with the blitzed seaweed. Combine the essential oils in a jug, then measure out 2.5ml (½ tsp) using a plastic pipette and add to the dry ingredients, stirring well to ensure they are fully mixed. Put the witch hazel into an atomizer and spray into the bowl until the ingredients seem slightly damp. Wearing vinyl gloves, check to see if the mixture clumps together when compressed in the hand; once this happens you are ready to place the mixture into the moulds.

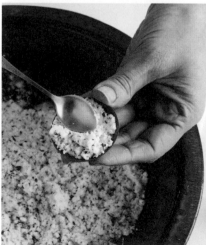

Step 2
Press the mixture into the moulds with the back of a teaspoon to ensure the powder is really compacted. Leave the moulds for at least 15 minutes to harden before inverting them on to a chopping board. Tap the base of the moulds to allow the tablets to drop down.

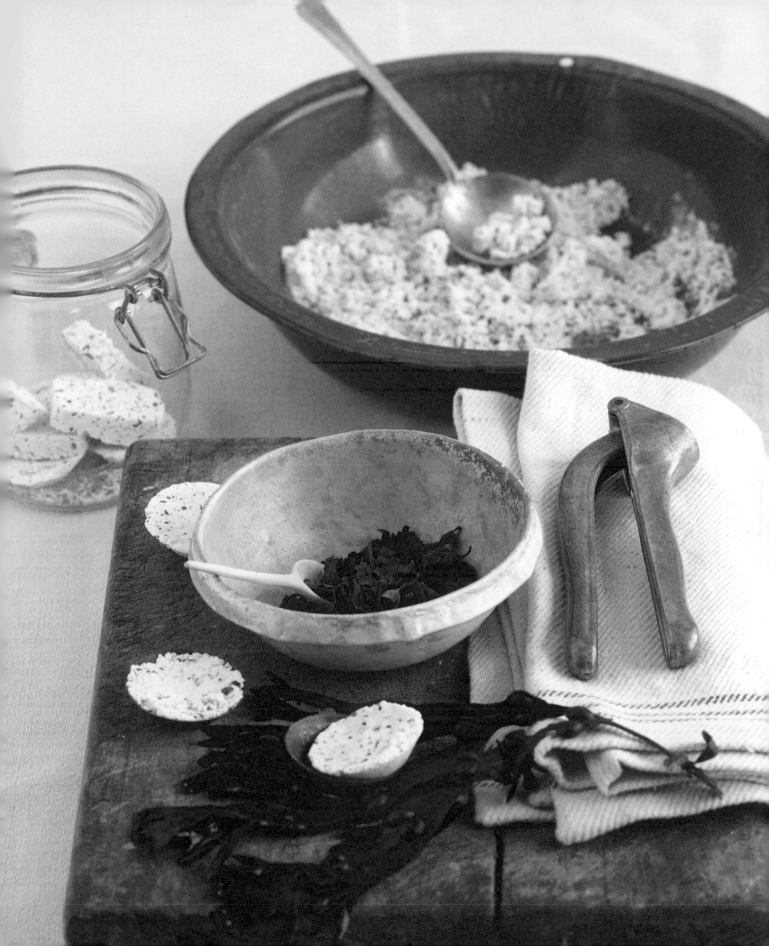

Shower Mud with Juniper, Cypress and Fennel

Why mud, I hear you ask? Well, once you've tried this unusual shower treatment combining clay and oats to both detox and nourish, you will see what we mean! It's spreadable, moisturizing and washes off like a milky body cleanser, leaving your skin feeling amazingly soft and supple.

Makes approx. 100ml (3½fl oz)

INGREDIENTS
10ml (2 tsp) Sucragel AOF
46ml (3 tbsp) sunflower oil
5g (1 tsp) oat flour or porridge oats
23g (¾oz) kaolin
10ml (2 tsp) Lamesoft PO65
5ml (1 tsp) glycerine
7 drops cypress essential oil
5 drops fennel essential oil
8 drops juniper essential oil

SPECIAL EQUIPMENT
plastic pipette
flat-bladed knife or palette knife

SAFE STORAGE
Ideally, the mud should be used straight away, but it will keep in a clean, sterilized jar in a cool, dry place away from sunlight for up to 3 months.

HOW TO APPLY
Apply to the body before showering, paying particular attention to areas of dry skin such as the knees, elbows and feet. The mud will dissolve in water and leave the skin feeling soft and moisturized.

Tip!
This recipe is a little more time-consuming than some of the others (although the extra effort is more than worth it!), so you could always make double the amount to save time at a later date.

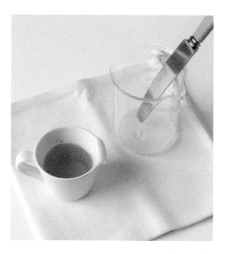

Step 1
Measure the Sucragel into a beaker and the sunflower oil into a jug. Using the pipette, add the oil to the Sucragel only a few drops at a time, to avoid the mix splitting, and blend with a knife. Use all the oil, which will make a firm gel; it will appear cloudy at first, but will become clear if left.

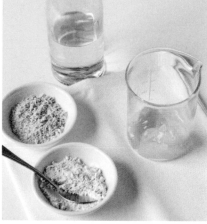

Step 2
If you are using porridge oats, these will need to be whizzed in a spice grinder or blender to form a fine powder. You may need to whizz the oats a few times to get a really fine, smooth powder. Add the oat flour to the kaolin clay in a bowl and mix to combine well.

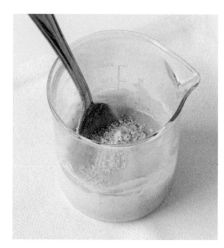

Step 3
Add the whizzed porridge oats and clay to the gel in the beaker, along with the Lamesoft PO65, the glycerine and the cypress, fennel and juniper essential oils. Use a metal spoon to mix well, until the mixture reaches the consistency of a spreadable mud.

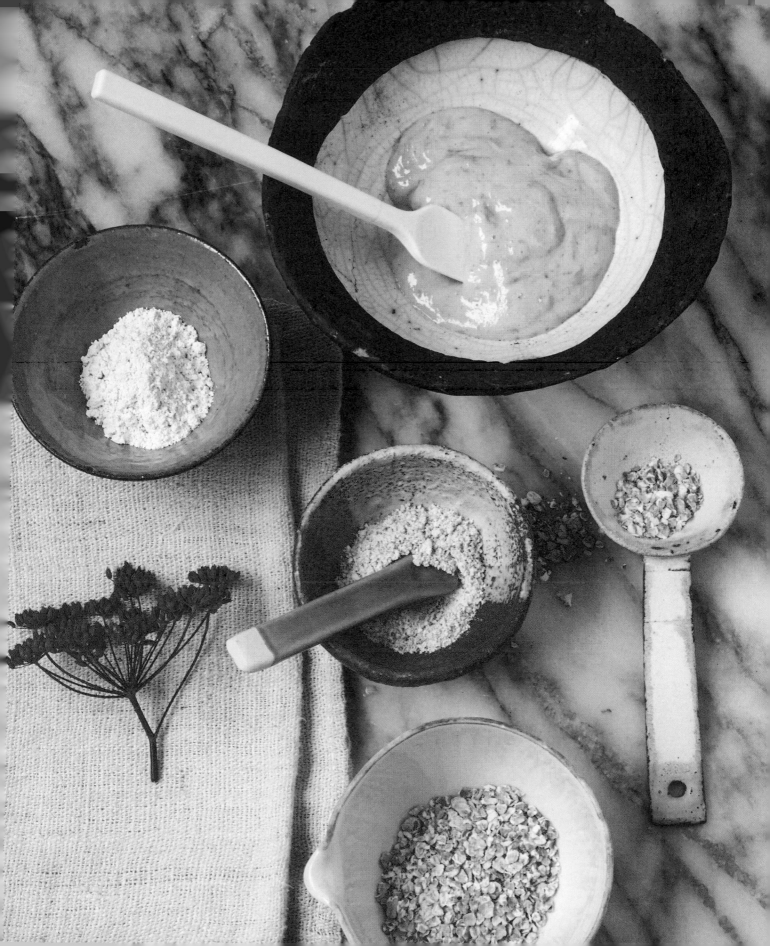

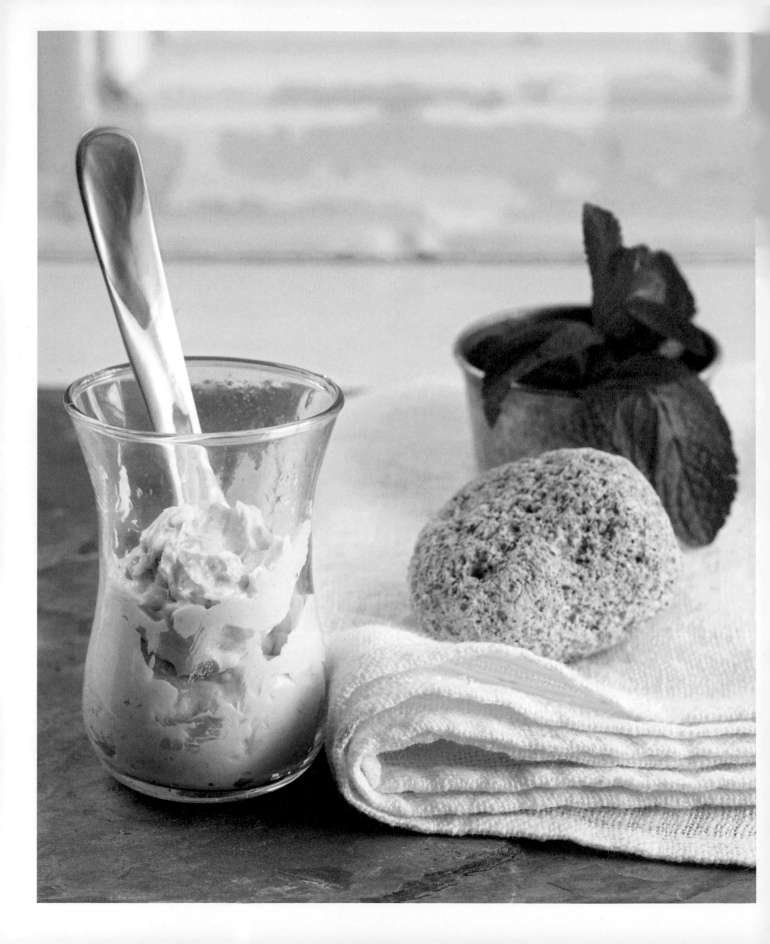

Creamy Foot Scrub with Peppermint and Pumice

This creamy scrub is ideal for exfoliating dead skin from the heels and feet, while giving your feet a moisturizing treatment at the same time. The fresh scent of peppermint, combined with lavender, cypress and lemon balm will leave your feet fresh and restored, ready to slip into those revealing peep-toe shoes or strappy sandals.

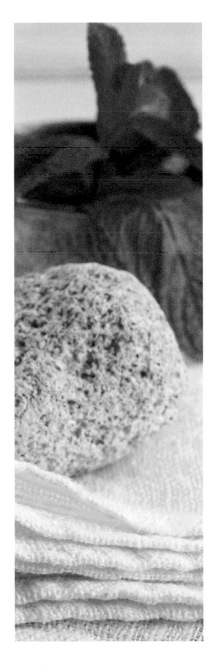

Makes approx. 100ml (3½fl oz)

INGREDIENTS
3ml (½ tsp) glycerine
58ml (2fl oz) peppermint water
3g (½ tsp) cetearyl alcohol
5g (1 tsp) Olivem 1000
5g (1 tsp) unrefined coconut oil
10ml (2 tsp) sweet almond oil
6g (1¼ tsp) shea butter
8g (1½ tsp) fine- to medium-grade
  pumice powder
5 drops lavender essential oil
5 drops cypress essential oil
5 drops lemon balm essential oil
40 drops grapefruit seed extract

SPECIAL EQUIPMENT
heatproof jug
metal saucepan
thermometer
stick blender
sterilized airtight glass jar and lid

SAFE STORAGE
Store in a cool, dry place, away from sunlight. Keeps for up to 3 months.

Step 1
Measure all the ingredients except the pumice, essential oils and grapefruit seed extract into a heatproof jug.

Step 2
Place the jug in a pan of simmering water and heat to 70–80°C (158–176°F). Maintain this temperature for 30 minutes, then remove from the heat.

Step 3
Whizz the mixture with a stick blender, then leave to cool to around 40°C (104°F). Add the pumice, essential oils and grapefruit seed extract, and stir to incorporate the pumice evenly. Spoon into a sterilized airtight jar and secure the lid once completely cool.

HOW TO APPLY
Massage the scrub into the feet, paying particular attention to the heels, toenails and any areas which have hard skin. Rinse and dry the skin.

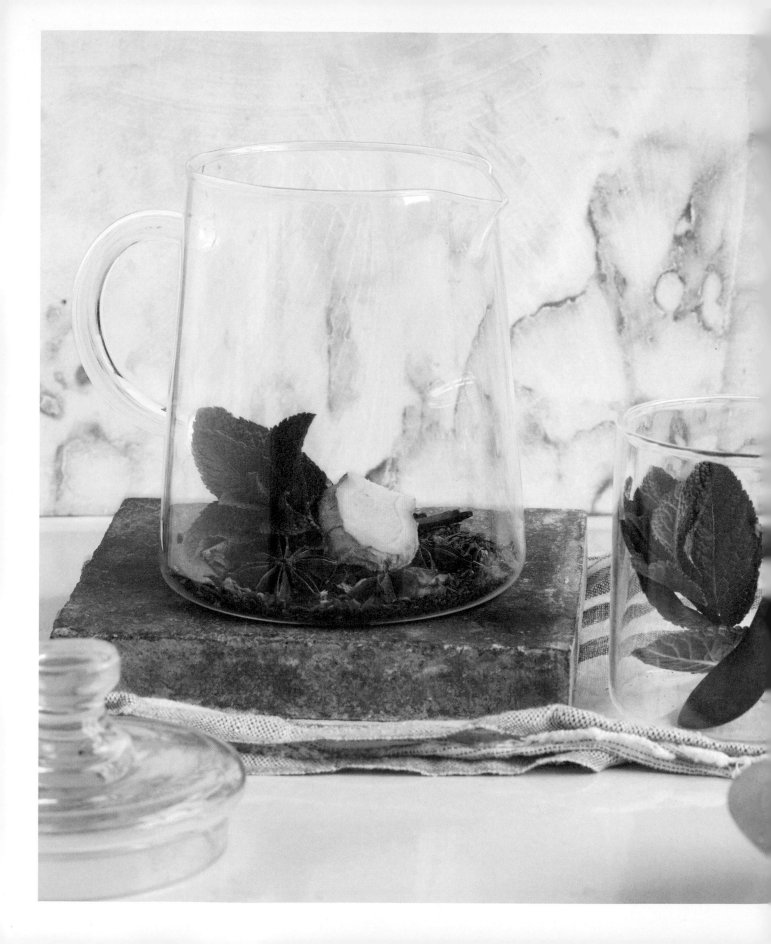

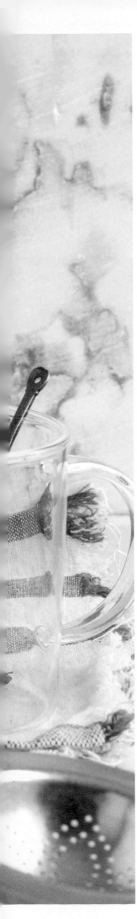

Herbal Detox Tea

It's easy to make your own herb-based teas using fresh ingredients from your garden or windowbox, augmented with some dried botanical ingredients from a supermarket, health-food store or online specialist (see Directory of Suppliers, page 142). A tea infuser or glass teapot with an infusing compartment will make you feel like a pro, but you can simply infuse your tea in an existing teapot or jug and use a tea strainer or small sieve for the same results. Using fresh mint leaves, especially peppermint, will greatly enhance the flavour and aroma of your tea, as well as increasing the detoxifying and digestive properties of the drink.

Makes approx. 2 cups

FRESH INGREDIENTS
few slices of root ginger
2 sprigs of peppermint or
    spearmint leaves, plus extra for
    the cup
optional: honey

DRY INGREDIENTS
15g (1 tbsp) loose-leaf
    gunpowder green tea
3g (½ tsp) chopped burdock root
5g (1 tsp) chopped liquorice root
2 or 3 pieces of star anise
1 cinnamon stick

SPECIAL EQUIPMENT
kettle
teapot or jug
2 cups, mugs or tea glasses
optional: tea strainer

SAFE STORAGE
The tea should be made fresh each time and consumed immediately.

Step 1
Pick your fresh ingredients, wash them if needed, then set aside.

Step 2
Measure out the dry ingredients into a bowl. You can make a larger amount and store it in an airtight tin or glass jar with a lid for later use; always label your jar so you know it is a tea mix.

Step 3
Place 1 or 2 teaspoons of the dry mix in a teapot or jug, along with the ginger and mint. Pour over enough hot water for 2 cups; the water must be hot (but not boiling) to avoid the green tea developing a harsh taste. Allow to infuse for 5 to 10 minutes before pouring into a cup or mug (through a strainer if you are not using an infusing teapot). You can also use a tea glass, but remember to place a metal spoon in the glass before pouring in the hot liquid to avoid cracking.

Step 4
Add a few more mint leaves to the cup. The amount of mint you use is optional, depending on how minty you like your tea. You can also add a teaspoon of honey to sweeten the tea, if you wish.

Tip!
The dry ingredients mix of this tea can be made and stored for up to 3 months. This will make the teamaking process quicker. Store the mix in an airtight tin, or glass jar with a secure lid.

Adaptation:

Camomile Tea Eye Pads

....

You may be fond of camomile tea, but you have probably never thought of using it as a spa treatment. However, the beneficial, restorative qualities of herbal teas make them ideal ingredients for eye pads or compresses, while camomile is soothing and calming to the skin. Choose herbal teas from premium brands where the ingredients used are bulkier whole leaves and flowers, as opposed to the fine powders which tend to be a feature of the budget teas.

INGREDIENTS
camomile flower tea bags (such as teapigs)

SPECIAL EQUIPMENT
cotton wool pads

Place a teabag in a cup or mug and pour over boiling water. Allow the tea to infuse and cool for around 10 minutes.

Dip a couple of cotton wool pads into the tea so they are soaked, and squeeze out the excess moisture. Check the pads are warm but not too hot.

SAFE STORAGE
The tea should be made fresh each time and used immediately.

....

HOW TO APPLY
Place the pads over closed eyes and lie back while the warming pads soothe and relax tired eyes.

Adaptation:

Green Tea Eye Pads

....

Green tea is another wonderful herbal tea option for using as soothing eye pads. It is an antioxidant and anti-inflammatory, which can offer anti-ageing benefits. The larger oval cotton wool pads are our favourites for this recipe as their shape is better suited to use around the eye area. We also like to use loose-grade green tea from specialist ethnic stores and health-food shops. Make the tea in a teapot, leave it to infuse fully, and then strain into a glass or mug to cool, as for the teabag option below.

INGREDIENTS
green tea bags (such as teapigs)

SPECIAL EQUIPMENT
cotton wool pads

Place a teabag in a cup or mug and pour over boiling water. Allow the tea to infuse and cool for around 10 minutes.

Dip a couple of cotton wool pads into the tea so they are soaked, and squeeze out the excess moisture. Check the pads are warm but not too hot.

SAFE STORAGE
The tea should be made fresh each time and used immediately.

....

HOW TO APPLY
Place the pads over closed eyes and lie back while the warming pads soothe and relax tired eyes.

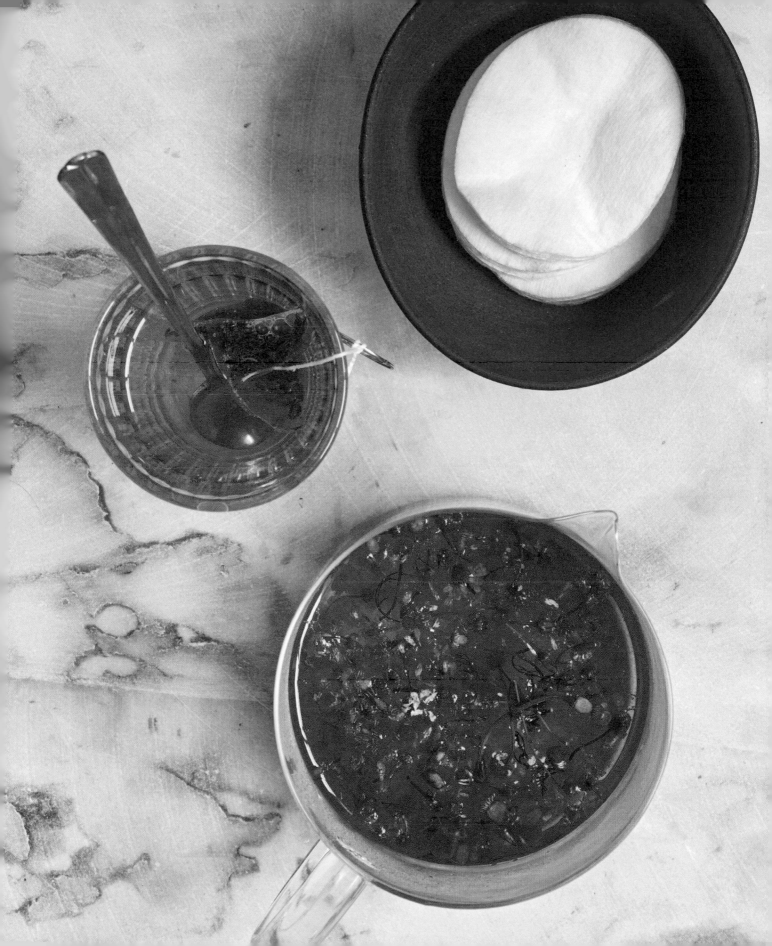

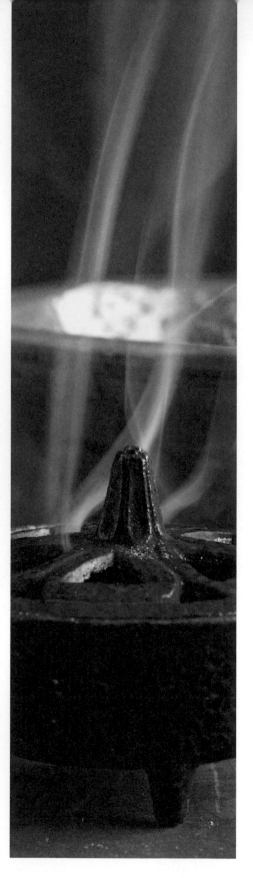

Purifying Incense Powder and Cones

The use of incense is centuries old and has its roots in many different parts of the world, from the master incense-makers of Japan to the Spice Road in India, the Christian churches in Europe and the origins of self-burning incense from China. Often bound up with religious practices, incense has a mystical quality and is believed by many to be a source of energy and capable of creating a sacred space. It is cleansing and can help with meditation – and if you really want to find a way to banish an unwelcome odour from your home, incense is the way to do it.

Making your own incense is a really satisfying task. You can keep it simple and assemble some wood powders, aromatics and herbs to make a loose powder for burning on a charcoal disc. Or you can experiment with creating specific blends which can be formed into cones and burned on their own, with no need for the assistance of heat from charcoal. This allows you to achieve a purer scent, which is entirely derived from the wood powder that you have chosen and doesn't have the familiar charcoal background odour.

As with our cosmetic recipes, your garden can be a source of inspiration for incense-making materials. Anything you use will need to be dried completely to allow it to burn, so it is a good idea to gather up leaves and even small herb and flower stems which can be dried in your airing cupboard and used later. Try some of the following ideas: scented pelargonium, lavender, cistus, pine tree resin, viburnum, thyme, rosemary, oregano, marjoram, salvia, juniper, peppermint. You could also raid your spice cupboard for cinnamon, clove, nutmeg, star anise. Remember that these materials are only used in loose incense (not cones) and must be ground to a powder prior to use.

Incense Powder

Loose incense is very simple to produce from a variety of dried materials and can be assembled and burned straight away. You can use a combination of the suggested ingredients below, or adapt the recipe to suit the materials that you have, and have fun experimenting using your own ideas.

INGREDIENTS
The best materials for loose incense are gums such as frankincense, myrrh, pine and rosin, available from online suppliers. You can also add powdered woods such as cedarwood and sandalwood, and dried herbs like lavender, rosemary and thyme. However, due to the heat of the charcoal, these botanical elements will tend to have only a fleeting effect as the smell of the charcoal woods and gums can overwhelm more delicate aromas.

5g (1 tsp) yellow sandalwood powder

5g (1 tsp) ground resin such as myrrh or frankincense

5g (1 tsp) dried botanical such as pelargonium or rosemary leaves

5g (1 tsp) spice powder such as cinnamon, allspice or nutmeg

15g (1 tbsp) makko

Mix all the ingredients together so they are well blended.

SAFE STORAGE
Store the powder in a cool, dry place, away from sunlight. Keeps for up to 12 months.

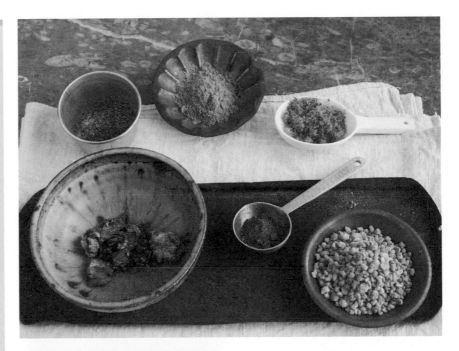

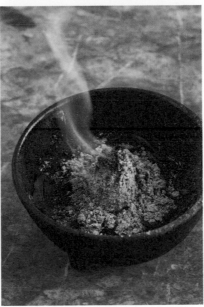

INSTRUCTIONS FOR USE

Step 1
Place a charcoal disc in a suitable incense burner placed on a heat-resistant surface. Light the disc with a long match. Ensure that it is alight and leave to burn until the disc has transformed from black to pale grey and is very hot. Do not touch the disc.

Step 2
With a metal teaspoon, carefully place a small amount of the powder on the lit disc and allow to burn. The aroma will gradually fill the room, although the powder will burn quickly.

Incense Cones

Makes approx. 20

INGREDIENTS

18g (3½ tsp) sandalwood
  powder, or other wood powder
  such as cedarwood
15g (1 tbsp) makko
1g (¼ tsp) cellulose gum binder
approx. 25ml (5 tsp) water

SAFE STORAGE
Store the cones in a cool, dry
place, away from sunlight. Keep
for up to 12 months.

Cone-making is simple, but it requires practice to achieve the right consistency of wet material, combined with the correct tapered shape which allows the cone to be lit and to burn evenly to the base. You will also need to allow several days for the cones to dry, so if you are in a rush, try the loose version first and plan to make the cones when you have more time.

Most shop-bought cone incense is made from unscented compressed blanks which have been dipped in fragrance, often from a cheap source. For this reason many people find incense unpleasant and overpowering. Making your own using naturally scented, unrefined ingredients is a totally different concept and immensely satisfying. The recipe here uses only natural plant materials so that the wood powder itself gives the scent to the room when burning.

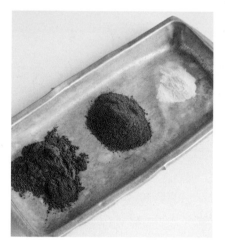
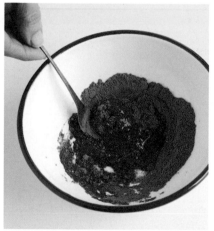
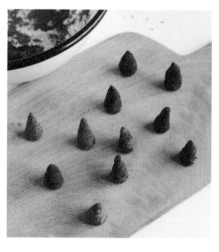

Step 1

Place the sandalwood powder, makko and binder into a bowl and mix together. Add the water gradually until you have a slightly wet, pliable dough. Pinch off around ¼ tsp of the incense dough and start to form the cones in the palm of your hand, by rolling the dough into a long cylindrical shape. You are aiming to get a pointed top and a flat base, which is best achieved by placing the rolled cylinder on a flat board or plate and pushing down gently so that it forms a stable base to the cone. The cones should be smooth without lumps or cracks in the surface. If the dough isn't wet enough you will notice the cone develops cracks which will prevent it from burning well, so if this is the case add more water to your mix and start rolling again. You can also mould the cones with damp hands, adding water as you roll them, which should enable you to smooth the surface as you go.

Step 2

Once you have rolled all the cones, place them on a plate to air-dry at ambient room temperature. Ideally, place them on their plate inside a large plastic box and cover with a lid for 24 hours, then remove the lid and let them dry naturally for 3 days. Resist the temptation to speed up the process by putting them somewhere hot – this will affect their ability to burn well. They should be totally dry to the touch and a lighter colour than when just made.

- If you wish to incorporate essential oils to your cones, add just 4 or 5 drops of your chosen oil at Step 1 along with the water. Essential oils are very powerful so add just a few drops per batch.

- If you have trouble getting your cones to burn, they are probably not dry enough. Leave them for another day or two and then try lighting them again.

- Many people don't seem to be able to smell sandalwood well, so if you find that your cones don't appear to have a strong scent, try using cedarwood powder instead.

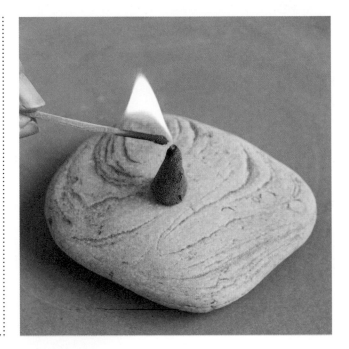

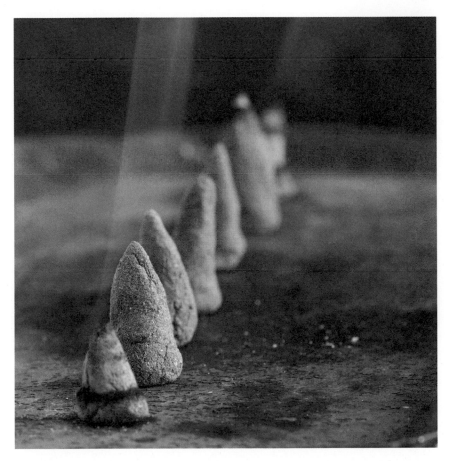

INSTRUCTIONS FOR USE

Step 1
To light a cone, place it on a suitable plate or other heatproof surface, as the cone will leave a resin residue after burning which is difficult to remove. We use a specific incense burner or a flat stone or pebble specifically reserved for incense.

Step 2
Light the tip of the cone and allow it to burn briefly. Generally the cone will self-extinguish after a few seconds; if it doesn't, blow out the small flame leaving a burning tip which will immediately give off a trail of smoke. If the incense cone stops burning altogether, try relighting it as sometimes it takes more than one go to get the cone burning correctly. The incense will burn for around 10 minutes, wafting the most amazing aroma around the room.

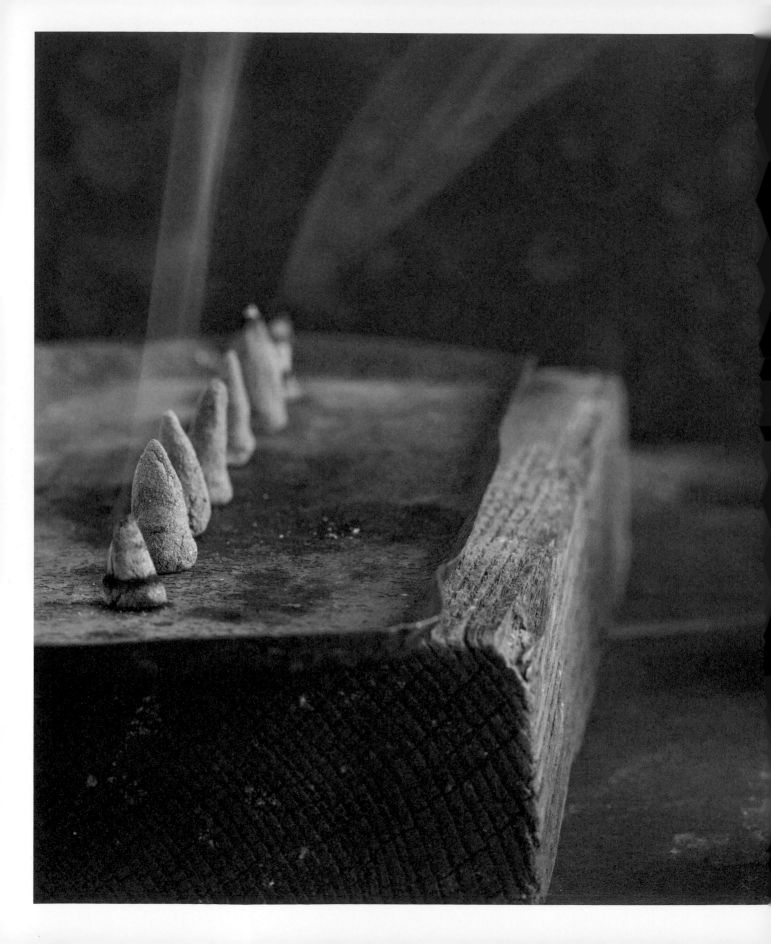

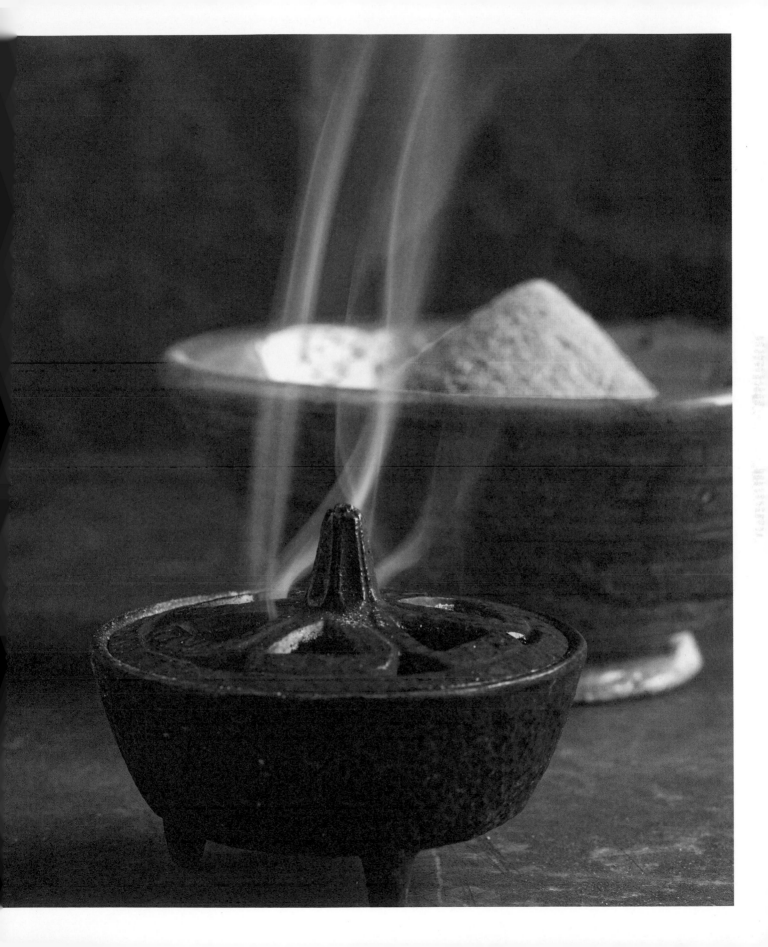

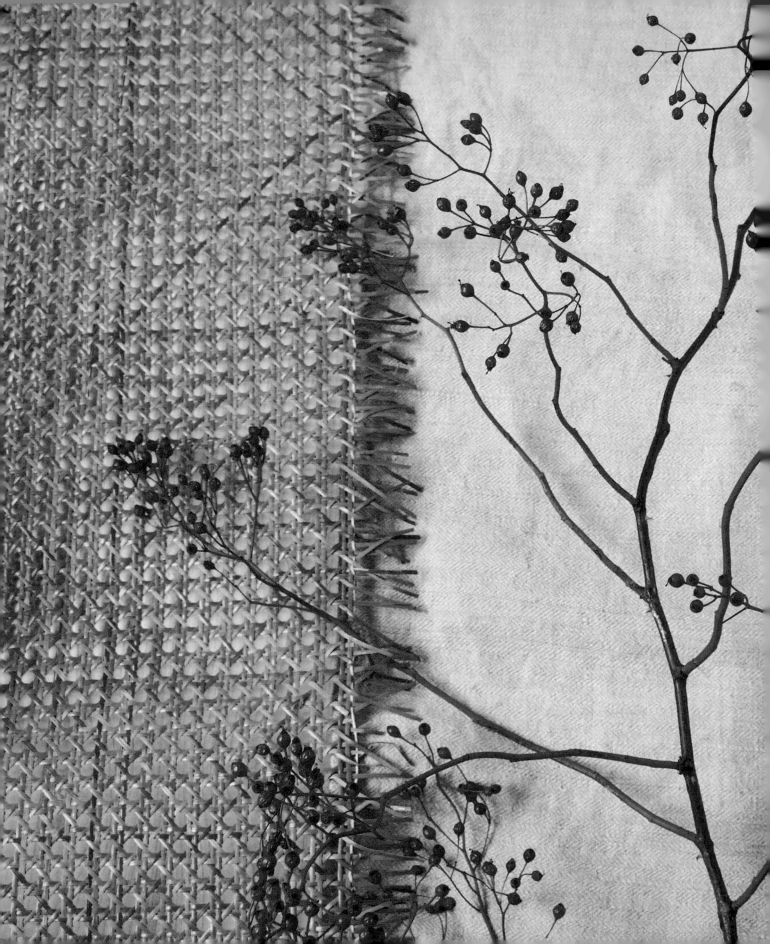

Glossary of Ingredients

Glossary of Ingredients

The following table includes all ingredients used in the book, their INCI name, and their health and beauty benefits. The cosmetics industry uses a common naming system known as the International Nomenclature of Cosmetic Ingredients (INCI). This means that the same ingredient names, based on scientific names, are used internationally, helping people to avoid the ingredients to which they're allergic.

KEY:
The symbols indicate where you will be able to buy the ingredients featured in the recipes in this book:

✚ CHEMIST (DRUGSTORE)
○ HEALTH-FOOD STORE
@ INTERNET
🛒 SUPERMARKET OR SPECIALIST SHOP

COMMON NAME	INCI (EU) NAME	BENEFIT
ALGINATE POWDER @	SODIUM ALGINATE, DIATOMACEOUS EARTH, CALCIUM SULPHATE	A natural polysaccharide product extracted from brown seaweed that grows in cold water regions. In the presence of calcium it sets to form a rubbery gel, making it ideal as a base for natural peel-off face masks.
ALOE VERA JUICE ○	ALOE BARBADENSIS LEAF JUICE	Great benefits in skin protection and repair; its soothing, cooling and healing effects are well documented.
AMYRIS ESSENTIAL OIL @	AMYRIS BALSAMIFERA BARK OIL	More commonly known as West Indian Rosewood or West Indian Sandalwood, and can be used as a cheaper alternative to genuine sandalwood. Amyris essential oil originates from Haiti and is often used as a perfume 'fixative' to extend the fragrant life of a blend due to its soft resinous aroma. It is also popular in aromatherapy for its grounding and soothing properties.
ARGAN OIL ○@	ARGANIA SPINOSA KERNEL OIL	Used for centuries by Berber women in Morocco to nourish their skin, hair and nails. Argan oil is exceptionally rich in natural tocopherols, carotenes, Squalane and essential fatty acids.

COMMON NAME	INCI (EU) NAME	BENEFIT
BAOBAB OIL @	ADANSONIA DIGITATA SEED OIL	This exquisite oil is cold-pressed from the seeds of the baobab fruit tree, known in Africa as the Tree of Life. The oil helps to improve moisture in hair and skin, stimulates the skin's recovery from external stresses, and enhances healing from within (hair and skin), instantly relieving dry, cracked skin. A natural source of vitamins A, D and E and Omega 3, 6 and 9 fatty acids.
BEESWAX WHITE BP @	CERA ALBA	The wax obtained from the honeycomb created by bees. It forms a protective barrier on the skin's surface, providing a shield against irritants while allowing the skin to breathe.
BENZOIN @	BENZOIN	A solvent extracted from resin of the Styrax benzoin tree that grows in Java, Sumatra and Thailand. It has a sweet, warm, vanilla-like aroma and has a calming and uplifting effect. Benzoin, also known as gum Benjamin, is one of the classic ingredients of incense and is also used as a fixative in the perfume industry.
BERGAMOT ESSENTIAL OIL @	CITRUS AURANTIUM BERGAMIA FRUIT OIL * must be bergatene/psoralen free *	The bergamot tree is common to South East Asia and also Italy. Bergamot oil is extracted from the rind of both ripe and unripe fruit by expression. The scent of the oil is basically citrus, yet fruity and sweet, and is used in aromatherapy for its uplifting effect. Bergamot oil often contains bergatene, which is sensitizing in the presence of sunlight, which is why the bergatene-free oil is recommended.
BURDOCK ROOT @	ARCTIUM LAPPA ROOT EXTRACT	A long tradition of use for its detoxifying and purifying health benefits. It can be found in supplement form or be eaten as a vegetable, and can also be made into a tea.
CAMOMILE TEA	CHAMOMILLA RECUTITA FLOWER EXTRACT	Camomile extract is renowned for many skincare benefits, including soothing and calming, plus radiance and brightening.

COMMON NAME	INCI (EU) NAME	BENEFIT
CEDARWOOD ESSENTIAL OIL ☺@	JUNIPERUS ASHEI OIL	Obtained from wood chips and sawdust of the North American cedar tree through steam distillation. It has a soft, clean, woody aroma and is known for its astringent properties, being beneficial for oily skin, acne and dandruff. It is also good for respiratory disorders.
CEDARWOOD POWDER @	JUNIPERUS VIRGINIANA	Cedarwood comes from several different trees known as cedars that grow in different parts of the world, and that have many uses from pencils to ship building. This red cedarwood powder is mixed from all parts of the tree and has a richer, more complex and uplifting scent and is ideal as a pure incense.
CELLULOSE GUM @	CELLULOSE GUM	Also known as carboxymethyl cellulose, this is a derivative of natural cellulose found in plant material such as wood and cotton. Cellulose is the most abundant organic polymer on earth. Cellulose gum is often used as a natural thickener and stabilizer for shampoos, creams and lotions.
CETEARYL ALCOHOL @	CETEARYL ALCOHOL	A mixture of fatty alcohols (cetyl and stearyl) derived from palm oil that takes the form of white flakes and is used as a co-emulsifier, emollient and thickener for creams and lotions.
CETYL ALCOHOL @	CETYL ALCOHOL	A fatty alcohol derived from palm oil that takes the form of white flakes and is used as a co-emulsifier, emollient and thickener for creams and lotions.
CHINESE GUNPOWDER GREEN TEA LEAVES ☺🗑	CAMELLIA SINENSIS LEAF	A classic green tea from China, made up of leaves hand-rolled into tiny pellets that resemble gunpowder, giving this tea its distinct name. Gunpowder tea is full-bodied with a hint of smokiness, and when blended with spearmint creates the famous 'Moroccan Mint' tea.
CINNAMON LEAF ESSENTIAL OIL ☺@	CINNAMOMUM CULILAWAN LEAF OIL	This warm, spicy oil is renowned for its distinctive aroma and antimicrobial properties.

COMMON NAME	INCI (EU) NAME	BENEFIT
CINNAMON STICKS 👌🧺	CINNAMOMUM VERUM	Rolled from the aromatic, spicy bark of tropical East Indian cinnamon trees.
CITRIC ACID 🧺	CITRIC ACID	A pH modifier.
COCO-GLUCOSIDE @	COCO-GLUCOSIDE	A mild, non-ionic, naturally derived and biodegradable surfactant. Recommended to create very mild and sulphate-free surfactant systems with good foam.
COCONUT OIL, UNREFINED 👌🧺	COCOS NUCIFERA OIL	This tropical oil has so many uses for skin and hair. Rich in fatty acids, triglycerides and natural tocopherol, it has excellent protective and moisturizing properties.
CORN STARCH @	ZEA MAYS	This fine powder is often used as a natural thickener or cosmetic powder base, imparting a smooth feel to the skin.
CRYSTAL CLEAR MELT AND POUR SOAP BASE @	GLYCERIN, AQUA, SORBITOL, SODIUM STEARATE, SODIUM OLEATE, SODIUM LAURATE	This vegetable-based, melt-and-pour soap base is made from 99 per cent natural ingredients and is free from surfactants. It produces natural translucent soap bars with good moisturizing properties due to its very high glycerine content, which also provides a pleasant skin feel.
CUCUMBER 🧺	CUCUMIS SATIVUS FRUIT EXTRACT	Renowned for its cooling and soothing effect on the skin.
CYPRESS ESSENTIAL OIL 👌@	CUPRESSUS SEMPERVIRENS OIL	This aromatic oil is obtained by distilling the small branches and leaves with steam. It is a venous decongestant, vasoconstrictor and has healing properties, particularly in the case of varicose veins.
DEMINERALIZED / DEIONIZED WATER 🧺	AQUA	A carrier, solvent and hydrator.
DISTILLED WITCH HAZEL BPC @	ALCOHOL DENAT; HAMAMELIS VIRGINIANA BARK/LEAF/TWIG EXTRACT	A renowned natural astringent, skin toner and skin refresher.

COMMON NAME	INCI (EU) NAME	BENEFIT
DRIED SEAWEED POWDER ⌂@	SPIRULINA MAXIMA POWDER	A well-known type of blue/green algae that can be found in the world's oceans and lakes. The vitamin-rich dried spirulina powder has antioxidant and detoxifying benefits for the skin.
EPSOM SALTS ✚⌂	MAGNESIUM SULPHATE	This amazing mineral has so many benefits. Easily absorbed by the skin, it helps to soothe and relax the body, relieve aches and ease muscular pains.
ESP ORGANIC SAFE-EMULS SCA @	ALOE BARBADENSIS LEAF JUICE; SUCROSE COCOATE	A unique combination of aloe vera extract with a natural emulsifier derived from coconut oil and sugar that has exceptional skin-softening properties, leaving it with a unique velvety feel. It enables oil and water to combine easily to form a stable cream.
EUCALYPTUS ESSENTIAL OIL ⌂@	EUCALYPTUS GLOBULUS LEAF OIL	This aromatic oil obtained from the leaves of the tree is anti-inflammatory, antimicrobial and has stimulating properties.
EVENING PRIMROSE OIL ⌂@	OENOTHERA BIENNIS OIL	This nutritious emollient plant oil is rich in essential fatty acids (EFAs) and gamma linoleic acid (GLA), which help to maintain the moisture barrier of the skin. It is ideal to help soothe and protect dry skin.
FENNEL ESSENTIAL OIL ⌂@	FOENICULUM VULGARE OIL	This aromatic oil distilled from the seeds of the plant has antimicrobial properties and is also helpful against cellulite.
FORMULATORS' ALCOHOL @	ALCOHOL DENAT; ISOPROPYL MYRISTATE; PROPYLENE GLYCOL	A special solvent/carrier blend based on alcohol, which allows the simple addition and blending of essential oils and fragrances to produce clear solutions. The volatile alcohol evaporates quickly as it is warmed by skin temperature to deposit the fragrance evenly, and gives a cooling sensation. It is also ideal for making diffuser oils.
FRACTIONATED COCONUT OIL @	CAPRYLIC/CAPRIC TRIGLYCERIDE	A fine emollient extracted from coconut oil that gives a light but silky skin feel without greasiness.

COMMON NAME	INCI (EU) NAME	BENEFIT
FRANKINCENSE ESSENTIAL OIL ☺ @	BOSWELLIA CARTERII OIL	Olibanum, also known as frankincense, is extracted from the tree resin and is known for its anti-ageing and skin-toning properties.
GERANIUM ESSENTIAL OIL ☺ @	PELARGONIUM GRAVEOLENS FLOWER OIL	This aromatic oil with its characteristic floral odour makes it ideal for skincare fragrancing. It also has antimicrobial and astringent properties, making it beneficial for natural deodorants.
GINGER ESSENTIAL OIL ☺ @	ZINGIBER OFFICINALE ROOT OIL	Extracted by steam distillation of the dried root. This warming essential oil has a strong, spicy, sharp aroma with a hint of lemon and pepper, and when topically applied it can relieve muscle aches and pains and poor circulation.
GINGER ROOT 🧺	ZINGIBER OFFICINALE	Common to India and China, this has many therapeutic properties, including relief from nausea and digestive problems, and is well known as a remedy for travel sickness. As a home remedy, it can be made into herbal tea to ease gut inflammation, boost liver health and to ward off colds, flu and sore throats.
GLYCERINE ✚ @	GLYCERIN	A highly effective humectant derived from palm oil that helps to maintain the moisture balance of skin and hydrate parched skin. It is one of the oldest and most respected moisturizers.
GRAPEFRUIT ESSENTIAL OIL ☺ @	CITRUS GRANDIS PEEL OIL	A zesty, refreshing aromatic oil extracted from the fruit peel. It has excellent cleansing properties and is ideal for oily skin.
GRAPESEED OIL ☺ @	VITIS VINIFERA SEED OIL	Has a very light skin feel, is easily absorbed and helps to reduce water loss.
GREEN CLAY @	ILLITE	French green clay has long been known for its detoxifying skincare benefits that can be attributed to its unique mineral composition. It helps to absorb skin impurities and is mostly recommended for oily, clogged or acneic skin.
GREEN TEA ☺ 🧺	CAMELLIA SINENSIS LEAF EXTRACT	Infusions of tea contain polyphenols that have antioxidant and anti-inflammatory properties, protecting the skin against damage that can be caused by free radicals. Also offers anti-ageing properties.

COMMON NAME	INCI (EU) NAME	BENEFIT
GROUND PUMICE @	PUMICE	These hard grains of volcanic rock make an ideal exfoliant for removing rough skin from busy, tired feet.
HOP ESSENTIAL OIL @	HUMULUS LUPULUS OIL	Famous throughout the world for flavouring beers, yet steam distillation of the flowers, known as cones or strobiles, yields a beneficial essential oil. The aroma is fresh and sweet with a sharp earthy and herbaceous aroma. It has sedative properties, hence its use in treatment for insomnia or sleeplessness. It is also beneficial for skin problems such as eczema, and improves the health of hair.
INCA INCHI OIL @	PLUKENETIA VOLUBILIS SEED OIL	This nourishing oil is a natural legacy from the ancient civilizations of Peru (the Incas), which has been carefully guarded until recently, and is extremely rich in Omega 3, 6 and 9 fatty acids. It is shown to be ideal for sensitive, damaged and dry skin and to have skin regenerative properties.
JASMINE ESSENTIAL OIL ♡@	JASMINUM OFFICINALE OIL	Originally from China and India, jasmine tea is a traditional Chinese drink. Solvent extraction of jasmine flowers produces a 'concrete' from which an 'absolute' is obtained by separation with alcohol. The essential oil is then produced off the absolute by steam distillation, and has a sweet, exotic and richly floral aroma with calming and soothing properties.
JUNIPER ESSENTIAL OIL ♡@	JUNIPERUS COMMUNIS FRUIT OIL	This aromatic oil is obtained from the needles, wood and fruit of the shrub. It has excellent antimicrobial and astringent properties.
KAOLIN @✚	KAOLIN	A soft white clay, commonly referred to as 'China clay', named after the hill in China (Kao-Lin) from which it was mined for centuries. It helps to draw impurities and toxins from the skin.

COMMON NAME	INCI (EU) NAME	BENEFIT
LABDANUM ESSENTIAL OIL @	CISTUS LADANIFERUS LEAF OIL	Steam-distilled from the crude gum obtained from the twigs of the *Cistus ladaniferus* shrub, or rockrose, that grows in southern Europe. It has a warm, sweet, herbaceous and musky scent, and has antiseptic and astringent properties. It is excellent for use in creams for mature skin to help to optimize a healthy complexion.
LAMESOFT PO65 @	AQUA; CITRIC ACID; COCO-GLUCOSIDE; GLYCERYL OLEATE; HYDROGENATED PALM GLYCERIDES CITRATE; TOCOPHEROL	Naturally derived from coconut oil and sunflower oil, it has positive moisturizing effects on the skin in surfactant/foaming cleansers.
LAVENDER ESSENTIAL OIL ♻@	LAVANDULA ANGUSTIFOLIA OIL	This multi-tasking aromatic oil has many skincare benefits due to its unique soothing and antimicrobial properties. It is also renowned for its relaxing fragrance and is ideal for night-time use.
LAVENDER FLOWERS ♻@	LAVANDULA ANGUSTIFOLIA	In Roman times the flowers were added to baths, which is where lavender gets its name (lavare means 'to wash'). The fragrant dried flowers give a pleasing visual texture and delicate fragrance to bath powders and body scrubs.
LAVENDER WATER @	LAVANDULA ANGUSTIFOLIA FLOWER WATER	The condensation biproduct from steam distillation of the essential oil. It has a delicate floral, herbaceous aroma and is an excellent tonic for the skin. Its calming and antimicrobial properties make it ideal for mild acne and for naturally cleansing the pores.
LEMON BALM ESSENTIAL OIL ♻@	MELISSA OFFICINALIS LEAF OIL	Steam-distilled from the melissa leaves and tops of the herbaceous plant, the warm and lemony aroma has calming and uplifting benefits. It also has antimicrobial properties and is excellent for refreshing tired and troubled skin.

COMMON NAME	INCI (EU) NAME	BENEFIT
LEMON ESSENTIAL OIL ⟳ @	CITRUS LIMON PEEL OIL	This fresh citrus aromatic oil helps to brighten and rejuvenate sagging or tired-looking skin. Its antimicrobial properties help to treat various skin disorders such as acne, and it is also recommended for reducing excessive oil on the skin. Also effective in hair tonics to help promote strong, healthy and shiny hair and eliminate dandruff.
LEMONGRASS ESSENTIAL OIL ⟳ @	CYMBOPOGON SCHOENANTHUS OIL	This characteristic lemony essential oil contributes to the fragrance of the product and has a mild deodorizing effect.
LIME ESSENTIAL OIL ⟳ @	CITRUS AURANTIFOLIA OIL	This mouth-watering citrus peel oil has antimicrobial properties and helps to fight acne and dandruff.
LIME POWDER @ 🧺	CITRUS AURANTIFOLIA PEEL	This fine zesty powder is made by grinding dehydrated lime peel. It offers gentle exfoliation and contains plant acids that help to cleanse and brighten the skin and even the skin tone.
LIQUORICE ROOT ⟳ @	ARCTIUM LAPPA ROOT EXTRACT	Liquorice has been used for many thousands of years to treat skin ailments. The root extract is renowned for its skin-soothing and skin-lightening properties.
LOOFAH ✚	LUFFA CYLINDRICA FRUIT	From the plant *L.aegyptiaca*, a member of the cucumber family. The fruit is allowed to fully mature and ripen, then dry out on the vine. The flesh then disappears, leaving only the fibrous skeleton and seeds, which can be easily shaken out to give the loofah that we know and use as a body scrub.
MAKKO @	MACHILUS THUNBERGII BARK	Makko or 'Tabu no ki' is the bark of the *Machilus Thunbergii* tree, cultivated mainly in South East Asia from Kyushu to China, Taiwan and Thailand. The bark is ground up and added to incense mixtures as a natural binder for making incense cones and sticks, and was first used as a replacement for sandalwood.

COMMON NAME	INCI (EU) NAME	BENEFIT
MANDARIN ESSENTIAL OIL @	CITRUS NOBILIS PEEL OIL	Extracted from the peel of the fruit by cold expression. It has a sweet and tangy aroma and complements other citrus notes for a refreshing effect. It is sometimes used to help to prevent stretch marks, while increasing circulation and reducing fluid retention.
MARJORAM ESSENTIAL OIL ⌖@	ORIGANUM MAJORANA LEAF OIL	Extracted from freshly dried leaves and flowering tops of the Mediterranean bushy herb by steam distillation. It has a warm, slightly spicy smell, and has calming, warming and relaxing properties, making it ideal for bath soaks to ease tired muscles.
MATCHA GREEN TEA POWDER ⌖@	CAMELLIA SINENSIS LEAF	A stone-ground powdered green tea used in traditional Japanese tea ceremonies. It contains small amounts of vitamins and minerals, but is most prized for being rich in the antioxidant polyphenol compounds catechins. Because matcha is made from ground whole tea leaves, it is a more potent source of catechins than standard green tea.
MEADOWFOAM OIL @	LIMNANTHES ALBA SEED OIL	A natural oil pressed from the seeds of white meadowfoam flowers, native to California, Oregon and British Columbia. The oil has a unique blend of fatty acids that gives it superior moisturizing and conditioning properties.
MELISSA WATER @	MELISSA OFFICINALIS FLOWER/ LEAF/STEM WATER	The condensation biproduct from steam distillation of the essential oil. Melissa water is an astringent and an ideal toner, tightening and awakening dull, sluggish skin while providing calming relief to the senses.
MINT WATER/PEPPERMINT WATER @ 🧺	MENTHA PIPERITA LEAF WATER	The condensation biproduct from steam distillation of the essential oil. This natural toner helps to keep your skin oil-free and fresh. It also helps to even skin tone and reduce puffiness around the eyes.
NEROLI ESSENTIAL OIL ⌖@	CITRUS AURANTIUM AMARA OIL	This uplifting essential oil from orange flowers can be used as a body perfume, and due to its potent antimicrobial properties is also beneficial for skincare.

COMMON NAME	INCI (EU) NAME	BENEFIT
OAT FLOUR	AVENA SATIVA	A fine powder of ground oats that helps to smooth and exfoliate the skin.
OLIVE OIL	OLEA EUROPAEA FRUIT OIL	Obtained from the ripe fruit of the olive tree. It consists primarily of the glycerides of linoleic, oleic and palmitic fatty acids and is reputed to help skin cell regeneration.
OLIVEM 1000 @	CETEARYL OLIVATE; SORBITAN OLIVATE	A natural 'PEG-free' emulsifier derived from olive oil that is easy to use and also has skin moisturizing benefits.
ORANGE ESSENTIAL OIL, SWEET @	CITRUS AURANTIUM DULCIS PEEL OIL	This essential oil is obtained from the peel of orange. It has a popular aroma and creates a happy, uplifted mood. It also has antimicrobial and cleansing properties and helps to brighten the skin.
ORANGEFLOWER WATER @	CITRUS AURANTIUM AMARA FLOWER DISTILLATE	Water produced from the distillation of orangeflower petals. This delicately fragrant water helps to soothe and refresh the skin.
PALMAROSA ESSENTIAL OIL @	CYMBOPOGON MARTINI OIL	This particular essential oil is popular in aromatherapy, as it has excellent skincare properties and a sweet uplifting rose-like odour. The oil is steam-distilled from the dry grass just before the flowers appear.
PEARL BARLEY	HORDEUM VULGARE	Pearl barley, or pearled barley, is barley that has been processed to remove its hull and bran, and it makes an ideal alternative to wheat for microwaveable 'hot packs'.
PEPPERMINT ESSENTIAL OIL @	MENTHA PIPERITA OIL	Contains menthol, which creates a cooling sensation that refreshes tired skin. It is also beneficial for oily skin. It is an excellent oil for rejuvenating the hair follicles, stimulating the scalp and promoting hair growth.
PEPPERMINT LEAVES @	MENTHA PIPERITA LEAF	Peppermint is native to Europe and is a cross between water mint and spearmint. Peppermint tea is delicious and refreshing and offers many benefits, including improving digestion, reducing inflammation and relaxing the body and mind.

COMMON NAME	INCI (EU) NAME	BENEFIT
PEPPERMINT WATER @ 🧺	MENTHA PIPERITA WATER	See 'Mint Water'.
PETITGRAIN ESSENTIAL OIL @	CITRUS AURANTIUM AMARA LEAF/TWIG OIL	Extracted from the fresh leaves and young and tender twigs of the orange tree through steam distillation. It is a popular perfumery ingredient, having an uplifting aroma, and is useful for deodorizing and skin infections due to its antimicrobial properties.
PLANTAPON LGC @	SODIUM LAURYL GLUCOSE CARBOXYLATE (AND) LAURYL GLUCOSIDE	A mild 'green' liquid surfactant blend which can be used to make up a base for foaming cleansing products such as shower gels, body washes, face washes, etc.
POLYSORBATE 20 @	POLYSORBATE 20	A solubilizer/emulsifier derived from sugar that enables the essential oils/oils/fragrance to mix in with an aqueous base.
POMEGRANATE OIL @	PUNICA GRANATUM OIL	Contains 'punicic acid', a unique Omega 5 fatty acid, which has strong anti-inflammatory properties. The oil helps to fend off free radicals keeping skin ageing at bay. It also provides skin regenerative properties and helps to protect against sun damage.
PORRIDGE OATS 🧺	AVENA SATIVA	Oats have many benefits for all skin types. They are very effective in addressing dry skin as they contain beta-glucan, which forms a fine protective film and penetrates to provide deep moisturization. They also have anti-inflammatory properties that are effective in healing dry and itchy skin. Oat flour will absorb and remove excess oil and bacteria from your skin and exfoliate dead skin cells, thus helping to combat acne.
PRESERVATIVE GSE (GRAPEFRUIT SEED EXTRACT) 🍏@	CITRUS GRANDIS EXTRACT	A bioflavonoid concentrate prepared from the seeds, pulp and white membranes of grapefruits. It is used as a broad spectrum, non-toxic, antimicrobial compound.
PUMICE POWDER @	PUMICE	The solidified lava from volcanoes. This natural material is commonly used in its raw state for smoothing rough skin on hands and feet.

COMMON NAME	INCI (EU) NAME	BENEFIT
RAPESEED OIL	BRASSICA CAMPESTRIS SEED OIL	Rapeseed, or canola, oil is extracted from the seeds of yellow flowering rape plants and has excellent emollient and protective properties for dry skin. Cold-pressed rapeseed is a natural source of vitamin E, a strong antioxidant which protects against free radicals that can damage and age the skin.
RICE BRAN OIL	ORYZA SATIVA BRAN OIL	An excellent natural, non-greasy emollient and moisturizer. It is rich in antioxidant vitamin E and gamma-oryzanol, protecting against free radicals and skin dryness.
RICE GRAIN	ORYZA SATIVA	Rice is the seed of the grass species Oryza sativa. This cereal grain is the most widely consumed staple food for a large part of the world's population, but it also makes an ideal alternative to wheat for microwaveable 'hot packs'.
ROSE GERANIUM ESSENTIAL OIL	PELARGONIUM GRAVEOLENS FLOWER OIL	This sweet and rosy essential oil is steam-distilled from geranium flowers, and occasionally leaves and stalks. It is often used in aromatherapy for its uplifting and balancing properties.
ROSEHIP OIL	ROSA CANINA FRUIT OIL	Rich in Omega 3 and 6, vitamin A and antioxidant tocopherols, this helps to protect, repair and restore the skin and maintain moisture balance.
ROSEWATER	ROSA DAMASCENA FLOWER WATER	The condensation biproduct from steam distillation of the essential oil. It adds a delicate fragrance to products and is an ideal toner for soothing irritated skin due to its anti-inflammatory properties.
ROSEMARY ESSENTIAL OIL	ROSMARINUS OFFICINALIS LEAF OIL	Regular use of rosemary oil helps to stimulate follicles, nourishes the scalp and removes dandruff. It is also believed that rosemary oil slows down premature hair loss and greying of the hair. It has antimicrobial properties and can help to tone the skin.

COMMON NAME	INCI (EU) NAME	BENEFIT
SANDALWOOD ESSENTIAL OIL ⏏@	SANTALUM ALBUM OIL	An essential oil obtained from the steam distillation of chips and billets cut from the heartwood of the sandalwood tree. The oil is known for its exotic, woody, sweet smell and is frequently used as a base for products such as incense and perfumes. It is also used in aromatherapy for its various benefits, including calming and harmonizing, and has antimicrobial properties.
SANDALWOOD POWDER @	SANTALUM ALBUM or Indian sandalwood SANTALUM SPICATUM or Australian Sandalwood	Sandalwood has always had strong links with many of the world's spiritual groups, and the powder can be burnt to produce a distinctive relaxing and meditative scent, and is commonly used in incense cones.
SEAWEED (SERRATED WRACK) @	FUCUS SERRATUS	This olive-brown shrubby seaweed contains natural antioxidant compounds that have long been known to have pronounced anti-ageing, skin conditioning, repairing and hydrating effects.
SHEA BUTTER @	BUTYROSPERMUM PARKII BUTTER	Has a unique fatty acid profile, such that it readily melts at body temperature, thus making it an ideal emollient for skin. It has a high content of unsaponifiables and is also a natural source of allantoin, which combined yield soothing and protective properties.
SODIUM BICARBONATE (BAKING SODA) ⏏🛒	SODIUM BICARBONATE	The natural mineral form of sodium bicarbonate is nahcolite. It is often found dissolved in mineral springs and can be used in natural cosmetic products to smooth the skin, cleanse and as a deodorant. The 'fizz' generated by a bath bomb is when this material combines with citric acid in the presence of water.
SPEARMINT ESSENTIAL OIL ⏏@	MENTHA SPICATA HERB OIL	Extracted by steam distillation of the flowering tops of the spearmint plant. It doesn't contain as much menthol as peppermint, and as such is not as cooling, but it does have antimicrobial properties.

COMMON NAME	INCI (EU) NAME	BENEFIT
SPEARMINT LEAVES ♻@	MENTHA SPICATA LEAF	Spearmint is a herbaceous perennial plant whose leaves contain many of the active ingredients and a high concentration of the scent and flavour. Its benefits are similar to that of peppermint but it has a sweeter taste.
SPRING WATER 🧺	AQUA	A natural source of water, containing minerals and trace elements to help to rehydrate the skin.
SQUALANE @	SQUALANE	A fine, light and non-greasy emollient derived from olive oil that gives the skin an amazingly soft feel and a natural bloom.
STAR ANISE ♻@🧺	ILLICIUM VERUM	A spice that closely resembles anise in flavour, obtained from the seeds of the star-shaped fruits that grow on the evergreen star anise tree, *Illicium verum*.
STEVIA ♻🧺	STEVIA REBAUDIANA LEAF/STEM POWDER	A sweetener and sugar substitute extracted from the leaves of the plant species Stevia rebaudiana. Known as the sweet honey leaf of Paraguay, the leaves have been used traditionally for hundreds of years in both Brazil and Paraguay to sweeten local teas and medicines. The active compounds of stevia are steviol glycosides (mainly stevioside and rebaudioside), which have up to 150 times the sweetness of sugar.
SUCRAGEL AOF @	AQUA; GLYCERIN; PRUNUS AMYGDALUS DULCIS OIL; SUCROSE LAURATE	This unique natural emulsifying blend combines plant sugars, coconut palm and sweet almond oils. It is kind to delicate and dry skin and leaves it feeling ultra-soft and conditioned.
SUCRAGEL CF @	AQUA; CAPRYLIC/CAPRIC TRIGLYCERIDE; GLYCERIN; SUCROSE LAURATE	This unique natural emulsifier blend derived from plant sugars and coconut palm oils is gentle to the skin and leaves it with an ultra-soft conditioned feel.
SUNFLOWER OIL 🧺	HELIANTHUS ANNUUS SEED OIL	Sunflower oil is cold-pressed from sunflower seeds and is light and non-greasy. It is beneficial to the skin, helping to reduce moisture loss and support the skin's barrier function.

COMMON NAME	INCI (EU) NAME	BENEFIT
SWEET ALMOND OIL @✛	PRUNUS AMYGDALUS DULCIS OIL	Protects and softens the skin. It is rich in essential fatty acids and vitamin E.
THYME ESSENTIAL OIL ⟳@	THYMUS VULGARIS OIL	This aromatic oil is extracted through steam distillation of fresh flowers and leaves. It has medicinal and antimicrobial properties and is effective against insect stings and bites.
VEGETABLE GELATINE POWDER ⟳@🧺	AGAR AGAR; CARRAGEENAN; PECTIN; XANTHAN GUM; GUAR; LOCUST BEAN GUM	Vegetable alternatives to the traditional animal gelatine, providing the 'jelly-like' texture that is ideal for refreshing face masks.
VITAMIN C ✛	ASCORBIC ACID	Pure vitamin C is renowned for its potent antioxidant properties. It helps to brighten the skin, reducing the appearance of age spots and other types of sun damage, and also boosts healthy collagen production.
VITAMIN E ✛	TOCOPHEROL	Found widely throughout nature, particularly in wheatgerm oil. It is an effective antioxidant and free radical scavenger, so helps to protect the skin from environmental damage. It has also been found to be beneficial in scar reduction and wound healing.
WHEATGERM OIL ⟳@✛	TRITICUM VULGARE GERM OIL	Readily absorbed by the skin, delivering a healthy infusion of vitamins, antioxidants, fatty acids and phytosterols. These nutrients help to moisturize and heal dry or cracked skin, and also help to prevent scarring. In particular, wheatgerm oil is a rich source of vitamin E, which helps to reduce skin damage, fight free radicals, support healthy collagen formation and maintain even skin tone.
XANTHAN GUM 🧺	XANTHAN GUM	Thickener/stabilizer naturally derived from corn sugar through a bio-fermentation process. Commonly used in foods.
YLANG YLANG ESSENTIAL OIL ⟳@	CANANGA ODORATA FLOWER OIL	This uplifting essential oil is extracted by steam distillation of the fresh flowers of the ylang ylang tree. It can help to maintain moisture and oil balance in the skin, keeping it hydrated and smooth, but is mostly used for its exotic fragrance.

Directory of Suppliers

UK

ABSOLUTE AROMAS

absolute-aromas.com

Specialist online supplier, with an extensive collection of essential oils. Also sells carrier oils.

Ships internationally

AMPULLA

ampulla.co.uk

Online packaging supplier, selling glass, plastic and aluminium containers for cosmetics and food. Offers an excellent selection, with pricing from a single item to bulk quantities.

Also has a European site: ampulla.eu

AROMANTIC

aromantic.co.uk

Online supplier of cosmetic ingredients, containers and kits. Also offers skincare and cosmetic courses in Scotland (where the company is based) and London.

Ships internationally

G. BALDWIN AND CO

baldwins.co.uk

171/173 Walworth Road, London, SE17 1RW

Retail store and online supplier of herbs, vitamins and supplements, as well as incense materials and burners. Also offers skincare courses in London.

Ships internationally

CANDLE SHACK

candle-shack.co.uk

Online supplier of candle-making equipment.

COMPAK SOUTH

compaksouth.com

Online supplier of glass containers. Specializing in food containers, but also sells clip-top jars, smaller bottles and jars, and closures for cosmetics, as well as a few plastic items.

GRACEFRUIT

gracefruit.com

Online supplier of cosmetic ingredients. Also stocks packaging, fragrances and flavours, and bases.

Ships to Europe

HAYES AND FINCH

www.candlewick-supplies.com

Suppliers of candle wax, candle wicks, cores and sustainers. Helpful website with tips on how to make and use candles.

HOLISTIC SHOP

holisticshop.co.uk

Online supplier of incense materials, herbs and supplements.

HOLLAND AND BARRETT

hollandandbarrett.com

Large chain of local health-food stores, located in most large towns in the UK. Sells food ingredients, including nuts, seeds and cereals, as well as essential oils, vitamins and supplements.

INCENSE SHOP

www.incense-shop.co.uk

Suppliers of blended incense and ingredients.

MISTRALNI

www.mistralni.co.uk

Supplier of formulators' alcohol.

NATURALLY THINKING

naturallythinking.com

Supplier of cosmetic raw materials.

PELL WALL

www.pellwall.com

Supplier of perfumery raw materials.

THE SOAP KITCHEN

thesoapkitchen.co.uk

Online supplier of a wide range of cosmetic ingredients, starter kits, and bath bomb and soap moulds. Also offers courses in making soaps, creams and bath bombs, as well as general technical advice.

Ships to Europe

USA

BRAMBLEBERRY

brambleberry.com

Online supplier of soap-making and other cosmetic ingredients, essential oils, moulds and packaging. Offers courses in soap-making.

Ships internationally

CANDLEWIC

www.candlewic.com
Suppliers of candle wax, wicks, moulds, as well as soap-making ingredients.

THE CHEMISTRY STORE

chemistrystore.com
Online supplier of soap-making and other cosmetic ingredients, equipment and packaging.
Ships internationally

FROM NATURE WITH LOVE

fromnaturewithlove.com
Online supplier of cosmetic ingredients, equipment, packaging and books.
Ships internationally

THE HERBARIE

theherbarie.com
Online supplier of cosmetic ingredients, packaging and books.
Ships to North America

MAKING COSMETICS

makingcosmetics.com
Online supplier of cosmetic ingredients, vitamins, fragrances, equipment, packaging and books.
Ships internationally

SCENTS OF EARTH

www.scents-of-earth.com
Suppliers of incense resins, herbs and woods, as well as incense mixtures.
Ships internationally

Australia and New Zealand

NEW DIRECTIONS

newdirections.com.au
Online supplier of essential oils, herbal extracts, cosmetic ingredients, cosmeceuticals, equipment, packaging; also stocks Australian specialities, listed as native botanical skincare.
Ships internationally

SOAP NATCH

soapnaturally.org
Online supplier of ingredients, particularly for soap-making, but also for cosmetics; also stocks moulds and stamps.
Ships internationally

Europe

AROMA ZONE

www.aroma-zone.com
French online supplier of cosmetic ingredients, natural extracts and essential oils, as well as packaging.

DRAGONSPICE

dragonspice.de
German online health-food supplier with some cosmetic ingredients.

HELENA COSMETICA

www.helenacosmetica.nl
Dutch supplier of cosmetic and perfumery raw materials.

JABONARIUM

jabonariumshop.com
Spanish online supplier of cosmetic ingredients, essential oils, fragrances and packaging.

JEAN PUETZ

www.jean-puetz-produkte.de
German online shop for cosmetic, perfumery and soap-making materials.

MANSKE

manske-shop.com
German online supplier of cosmetic ingredients, essential oils and equipment.

URTEGAARDEN

www.urtegaarden.dk
Online supplier of cosmetic raw materials in Denmark. Also offers recipes and courses.

Acknowledgements

We would like to thank everyone at Jacqui Small for asking us to write a follow-up to *Handmade Beauty*, and to the amazing job they have done in sending our previous book all over the world. We are truly amazed at how far it has travelled, and the way that so many people in other countries have taken to making our recipes and telling us about them.

Our special thanks go to our lovely editor Rachel Malig with her all-important eye for detail, as well as Amanda Heywood for once again producing such fabulous images that leap out from the page and make you really want to make the recipes. Thanks are also due to Caroline Davis who works such magic with everything she touches. It goes without saying that we couldn't do this without you all!

Juliette: Thanks once again to Abi for her exceptional knowledge of cosmetic products and in particular for her tireless work on the glossary. Thanks to James Debnam for his help with the scented candles, and to Anny Evason, Julia Fogg and Barbara Fredriksson for their incense material foraging. Thanks to all those who bought *Handmade Beauty* and whose enthusiasm for it encouraged us to work on another book.

Abi: Many thanks to Juliette for her continued enthusiasm and energy throughout the project, and I echo my thanks to all who purchased our first book, *Handmade Beauty*. A special thanks to my late partner Anthony for his encouragement and support at the start of this book, and who sadly will not see it completed, and also thanks to my new canine friend Santa for his cheerful distraction.

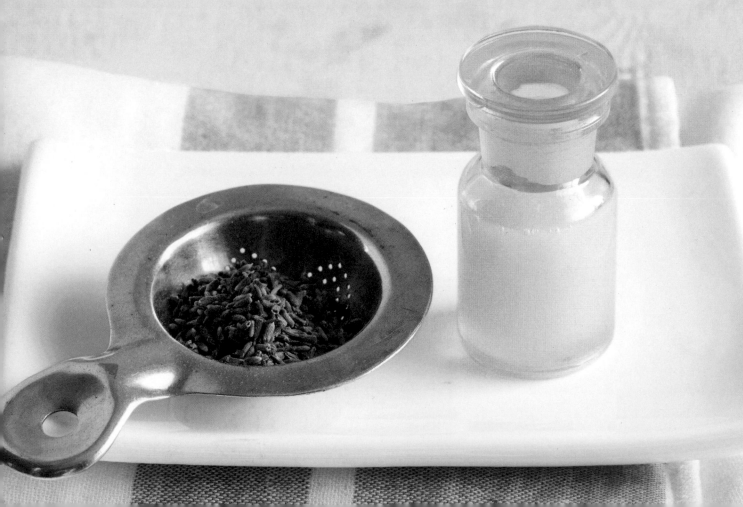